Carola Lemne

Handbook for Clinical Investigators

MW01229144

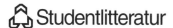 Studentlitteratur

Copying prohibited

Art.No 7223
ISBN 91-44-01301-9
© Carola Lemne and Studentlitteratur 1999
Translated by Carola Lemne
Cover art: Kjeld Brandt

Printed in Sweden
Studentlitteratur, Lund
Web address: www.studentlitteratur.se

Printing/year	1	2	3	4	5	6	7	8	9	10	03	02	01	2000	1999

Contents

Introduction

The term "clinical trials" is used for all the prospective studies of drugs or medical devices that are intended for investigating and demonstrating the efficacy and/or safety of drug therapies and other methods of medical treatment. The carrying out of clinical trials has become increasingly formalized in recent years. Governmental authorities have passed legislation, ordinances and guidelines; pharmaceutical companies have introduced formal "Standing Operating Procedures"; and most recently international – indeed, global – guidelines for "Good Clinical Practice" have been established.

This has occurred not simply due to demands from governmental authorities, but mainly because all the parties involved have come to realize that conclusive and high-quality study results can only be achieved through careful and consistent planning and execution. The discipline necessary for clinical drug trials is just as necessary and useful for all other types of clinical research projects.

This handbook is intended as an aid for "investigators" (that is, certified physicians and dentists) and others, prior to participating in any type of clinical trial, although it emphasizes drug trials.

1 General

Some background facts

Throughout the world thousands of drug trials are performed every year. Even if a large number of these concern new strengths or indications for existing drugs, or even generic preparations; a considerable number of studies concern completely new substances. Clinical trials have been performed to varying degrees for each new drug, preparation and indication. For drugs intended for long-term use in commonly occurring diseases, such as hypertension, it is not uncommon today for several thousands of patients, each treated for a year or more, to be included in the database submitted for registration.

This means that the number of clinical trials has also steadily increased, and this has been observed all over Europe, the US and also increasingly in other parts of the world. As an example there were slightly over 1000 applications to start clinical trials submitted to the Swedish National Board of Health and Welfare in 1982. In 1990 the corresponding number was nearly 1770 and in 1995 it passed 2200. Of these applications several could concern the same study; that is, more than one physician was involved in the same trial. This type of study, a multi-center trial, has become increasingly common; 1995's applications in Sweden involved just over 550 different studies, of which about 200 were international. There are no exact statistics on how many patients were included in all these trials, but an approximate estimate indicates that in Sweden alone more than 20 000 patients (and healthy volunteers) participated in clinical studies in 1996!

All medical disciplines are represented in clinical trials. The largest number of trials (just over 25%) involve internal medicine. This is followed by outpatient care, where an increasing number of trials are performed, and next comes general surgery. Trials are being run in private practice and in company employee clinics. Since the begin of 1995, the same standards have begun to be placed on medical devices as those already existing for drugs. This means that medical/technical products, such as infusion pumps, must be tested and documented in a similar fashion to drugs; that is, by performing clinical trials. In short, each physician and nurse can therefore count on encountering this phenomenon in his or her workplace at some time.

Clinical trials – Some definitions

The development of new drugs follows a given pattern, albeit with some variation. First comes the pre-clinical stage, beginning in the laboratory when possible new drugs are developed, these days often based on advanced knowledge about the body's cellular functions. Promising substances from *in vitro* experiments then enter an extensive animal-studies phase. This is partly an attempt to investigate the substance's possible effects, and partly to study the safety profile. Should the desired effects occur, the required toxicity studies are begun in order to eventually test the substance in humans. There are now harmonized guidelines for what to do and at times even in what sequence.

Once the pre-clinical program has advanced so far that there is an understanding about the substance's properties – both positive and negative – applications are submitted to regulatory authorities and to ethical committees for carrying out the first tests on humans; that is, to begin clinical trials.

Clinical trials are defined as a systematic administration of drugs (this includes common drugs, radioactive drugs, natural and related remedies, and some preparations for external application), or use of a medical device for the purpose of discovering or confirming their efficacy, patterns of adverse effects, pharmacokinetics, etc.

Clinical drug trials are usually classified into four different main phases, which have different purposes and characteristics:

Phase I comprises the first trials on humans. These are performed on healthy volunteers and are mainly intended to establish the tolerable dosage interval for humans. The investigations also study if and how the drug is absorbed, metabolized and excreted from the body. If possible, an attempt is also made to measure any effect, but since healthy volunteers are normally used in Phase I studies, this isn't always possible. One exception from using healthy volunteers in Phase I may be with trials involving cytotoxic drugs. Naturally, it is not advisable to administer these drugs to healthy volunteers – instead an opposite approach is used, the drug is administered to gravely ill patients who have been previously treated but without success.

If the Phase I studies show that the substance may be given to humans in reasonable doses and without overly troubling adverse reactions, Phase II generally follows. These are the first studies on patients having the disease intended for treatment and are meant to discover the minimum and maximum effective dose. The purpose is to extensively investigate how the drug behaves in the patients' bodies, which effects can be measured, and how these effects relate to a given dose, and so on. As mentioned above, these studies are performed on patients having the disease of interest, and an effort is generally made to enroll as homogenous patients as possible. Because there is uncertainty about the drug's possible effects, it is desirable to hold the number of possible confounding factors to a minimum. Consequently, it is highly desirable to have as "healthy" patients as possible (apart from the disease of interest) and who resemble each other as much as possible. In this way it is easier to discern the possible beneficial effect of the drug itself. Once Phase II is completed, there should be a good understanding about the drug's effects, suitable doses, and a preliminary understanding about the adverse reaction profile.

Phase III follows. Phase III studies are designed to document the drug's effects and adverse reaction pattern in "normal" patients. These studies include patients of various ages, patients with concurrent diseases, patients who are taking concurrent medication etc. Phase III is often divided into Phase IIIa and Phase IIIb. Phase IIIa are those studies that are to be included in the registration documentation, while Phase IIIb are studies that are performed prior to registration but are not included in the registration application. For example, these can be studies performed in order to conform to the treatment practices of different countries or to investigate special groups of patients. Once the Phase III program is complete, it is possible to begin talking about the drug's properties and common side-effects in a relatively representative cross-section of patients with some certainty; and the necessary documentation for getting the drug registered should now be available.

However, the drug's development does not stop once the drug is registered and permission to market is obtained. There often follows several years' of research in Phase IV studies. These are studies in which the registered drug is used for the registered indications using a registered dose. For example these studies can be large studies designed to discover rare adverse reactions (called Post Marketing Surveillance Studies), they can be studies that are designed to discover more mechanistic properties, or they can be long term mortality studies, such as those large cardiovascular studies that investigate the effect of anti-hypertensive drugs in preventing myocardial infarction.

It may be worth pointing out that if a registered drug is being investigated for another indication than the registered one, or using a new dosage, it is actually a Phase III, or even a Phase II study.

Clinical trials – why?

Clinical trials are required in order to register a drug, and also these days to obtain permission to sell various medical devices. They have the purpose of documenting the efficacy and safety of drugs and treatment methods that may some day be administered to thousands of patients. Physicians have a responsibility for their patients' health and included in this is the responsibility that the treatment methods used have a documented efficacy and safety. Participation in evaluating these new therapies and treatment methods ought thus to be an integrated part of all medical practice.

However – participating in clinical trials is sometimes boring, often puts one's patience to the test, and always involves more work than initially imagined. What makes a doctor become an "investigator"?

Being involved in a clinical trial often gives pure professional satisfaction. The physician gains more in-depth knowledge in the current topic and an opportunity to establish contact with other colleagues interested in the field. He/she keeps better up-to-date with developments in the field. The publication of the results can lead to valuable merits – and the opportunity to present the results at congresses that he/she might possibly not have been otherwise able to attend. "The trial" – the study – can often be a stimulating interruption in the daily routine and often creates the opportunity to have a more in-depth contact with the patients involved. In addition there are happy "side-effects" such as well-organized and productive project meetings during the study – and naturally the economic compensation for the extra work put in.

Regardless of the reasons put forth for participating in a clinical trial, the most important question remains "Do I personally feel that this study could be of use to the patients or for understanding the medical problem under consideration?"

If the answer is "no" it is perhaps wisest to refrain. Clinical trials entail so much effort in themselves that exclusively economic motives are often insufficient for keeping alive the personal motivation that is needed for obtaining qualitatively good results. Clinical trials require thoroughness to all details throughout, and the temptation to take a shortcut can be substantial if there is no genuine interest in the results.

There is often a sponsor behind a clinical trial. A sponsor may be a pharmaceutical company, a research fund or some other unit that has an interest in having a specific trial performed, and which supports the trial in various ways, e.g., economically. There are various reasons why a sponsor wants to conduct a clinical trial. It is always a question of evaluating some form of treatment, but the studies may have different formats depending on the sponsor.

Clinical trials sponsored by pharmaceutical companies are often designed to produce the necessary documentation for demonstrating the drug's efficacy and safety, and are required in order to get the drug registered. In addition, they often concern expanding the knowledge of an already registered drug – such as new indications, for example.

Clinical trials sponsored by authorities, funds or academic institutions can focus on evaluating treatment that lack commercial promise or methods that have been long used, but have never been thoroughly investigated before. One special area is research on drugs that are so old that the patent has long since expired. These drugs are commonly sold by generics companies that do not have the resources for, or maybe even interest in, further research on the substance. Such drugs are often called "orphan drugs," and it is precisely these substances that authorities and large institutions may have a need to investigate.

Regardless of the type of clinical trial in question, it is the doctor's commitment that matters. It is the physician who determines whether the study may be practical to perform at the clinic. The physician decides which patients are suitable, and the physician is a guarantor for the patients' welfare and integrity in the clinical research. Finally, it is also the physician who, with his/her own name, carries the responsibility for the reliability of the results.

Is there room for clinical trials within ordinary health care?

There is often a heavy workload in today's health care, and it may feel impossible to find the time for clinical research and clinical trials. While it is often officially said that continuous evaluation and verification of new treatments are a part of a physician's normal duties, the reality is that there is rarely time set aside for this. Participation in clinical trials requires careful advance preparation as well as consultation with superiors, colleagues and other coworkers who may become involved.

Talking with patients in connection to clinical trials usually takes more time than required when doing regular rounds or visits, especially in the beginning of the study when the project is to be explained and walked through. The time invested initially in carefully explaining the entire project is later paid back by having more enthusiastic and careful patients who more rarely withdraw from the study. Thus, this is time well spent, and it is important therefore to plan for this time right from the start.

In connection with their examinations, the patient often has many more questions than usual for the nurses and staff, and thus additional time may need to be reserved to cover this. Specially trained and hired nurses with research experience are invaluable in this respect!

Participating patients may experience suddenly appearing complaints, or get other diseases that may make it necessary to discuss the treatment with the physician responsible for the study. Thus, it is necessary to be prepared for the fact that additional work may occur outside of normal working hours.

In addition, the additional time required for updating patient charts, meeting sponsors and any other investigators, complementing missing data and a vast number of small but time-consuming details very often can only be attended to during leisure time.

However, careful review and planning can make it possible to handle these demands during the physician's allotted working hours – and thereby allowing not only the study to be performed, but also assuring high quality results.

Good Clinical Practice

Good Clinical Practice (GCP) is a term coined for labeling a collection of recommendations, rules and guidelines about how good clinical research ought to be performed. Thus, it is really a matter of Good Clinical Research (or "Trial") Practice. The phenomenon is exceptionally international. The FDA (Food and Drug Agency – USA) was the first to issue these kinds of rules and guidelines back in the 1960s. These guidelines are incorporated in US federal law, and violation of these can lead to prosecution – and although it rarely occurs, it remains fully possible. In England the pharmaceutical industry formulated its own guidelines, which were voluntary. The

French health care ministry issued guidelines in 1987 that later were incorporated into law and encompassed both Good Clinical Practice and a system for verifying that compliance to the law actually occurred. The European Union (EU) established a commission that worked out guidelines applicable to the entire EU and which were first issued in May, 1990. These guidelines are currently being reviewed and are planned to be issued in 2000 as directives; and thus become mandatory and not just guidelines. Other nations inside and outside of EU – such as Hungary – have however already chosen to incorporate GCP into law. Japan has produced similar guidelines and WHO has also released guidelines intended for use outside the USA, Europe and Japan.

Work began several years ago to further harmonize the US, European and Japanese guidelines. This work is being carried out within the framework of a large international cooperative forum under the collective name of "International Conference of Harmonization" (ICH). The aim is to arrive at an agreement about what documentation is needed for drugs (and to a certain degree also medical devices), both during the development phase in order to get the drug registered, and for ongoing monitoring of drugs on the market. In this way research need not be unnecessarily duplicated, and a universal and high standard will be obtained for all nations. A consensus has already been reached for some aspects, however there remains much work before drug research and development can be carried out and documented on a truly global basis. However, one of the aspects that has come far along in its development is specifically GCP. The ICH guidelines for GCP, ICH-6, has completed the entire process, were made official in May 1996, and are applicable to all clinical trials begun after January 1997 within ICH's jurisdiction, i.e. the US, EU and Japan. The new EU directive is built upon these guidelines, and work has begun in Japan to revise Japanese law in order to conform to ICH-6. The US authorities have previously made several changes, and at the time of this writing it is not certain whether additional changes are still to come. Given this abundance of guidelines, it is easy to wonder which ones actually apply. In the future it is intended that the ICH GCP guidelines are to be the basis for fundamental legislation – such as EU directives – which in turn will be mirrored in each country's own legislation. Minor local differences can sometimes appear, as they do already. Should differences between the two remain, it is the national legislation that applies, with the ICH GCP guidelines a solid second.

The same principles apply to the clinical testing of medical devices as for clinical drug trials. This is regulated within the EU by two directives

(93/42/EEC, MDD; 90/385/EEC, AIMD) These describe concepts so similar to the GCP used in clinical drug trials that the concept of GCP can be applied more or less equally to such activities as drug trials and evaluations of treatment methods or medical devices of various kinds. However, there are some differences concerning documentation, time allocated for official processing, etc. These differences will be specifically discussed in the appropriate chapters below – if nothing specific is stated, the described procedures are applicable for both drugs and medical devices.

GCP has several purposes. The two principal ones are protection of the patient's own self-interest, and to establish that clinical research be correctly carried out using high standards of quality and in such manner that it may be verified afterwards. The patients' own interest is primary, and their safety and integrity are (among other actions) protected by emphasizing the ethics committees' role and making them strictly obligatory. The content and quality of the information given to the patients is of very central significance. In addition there are detailed instructions about how adverse reactions are to be collected and reported. Both quality and verification functions are ensured via instructions on how the study project is to be set up, how data is to be gathered, verified regularly, and then stored for any later inspection.

Since the ICH collaboration, the various rules are steadily approaching harmonization. The US and EU requirements have previously differed on a number of points, but these are now far fewer in number and usually have no significant practical implications. However, in some cases, special requirements can appear that necessitate compliance with all the FDA directions. For example, this may occur when the drug being tested is manufactured and exported directly from the USA. According to US federal legislation, no drug may be exported for investigative use if US-federal regulations are not adhered to when the drug is later used. Considerable discussion may arise in these cases, since local legislation and directives are not always in complete agreement (see, "IND studies"). How this is to be resolved should be discussed with the sponsor on a case-to-case basis.

2 Sponsors

The investigator's responsibility

An investigator is the medicallyresponsible person (doctor or dentist) who takes a personal responsibility for carrying out the study according to the applicable directives and who ensures that the correct therapy is administered to all patients enrolled in the project.

Just what is it that an investigator takes responsibility for in connection with a study or clinical drug trial?

First and foremost it is the responsibility for both the patients' well-being and that the treatment being offered is the most appropriate in any given case. In order to ensure this, there are a great many things that are the investigator's lot throughout a study:

- To begin with, the investigator must be certified and well-merited within the field being studied (this applies to the person bearing the ultimate responsibility at each participating clinic; other coworkers at the clinic are not required to be have the same degree of specialist knowledge). The investigator must have good research skills and be familiar with all that is generally required in clinical trials (like GCP) and especially with the drug being investigated. The investigator is also responsible for ensuring that the resources needed actually exist. Investigators are often requested to prove their suitability via an attested curriculum vitae.
- The investigator must be knowledgeable of the drug or medical device under investigation (see "Investigators Brochure") and have good knowledge about the contents of the trial protocol. It is formally the investigator's responsibility to ensure that the trial protocol holds all the necessary information for designing and carrying out the study (see "The Study Protocol).
- The investigator must ensure that the personnel and equipment are adequate for taking care of the patients, and that the personnel are well

informed about the trial and procedures to be followed in any acute situation. The investigator must also inform and receive approval from the head of clinic, or the equivalent if applicable, and to make sure that no other projects are going on that can disturb the course of the study.

- One of the investigator's most important responsibilities is of course the information to patients and that the enrollment (or "inclusion") of patients is carried out in an ethically correct manner (see "Patient information and informed consent"). The patient's personal physician, or the equivalent, must also be informed that the patient is participating in the study if the patient is in agreement with this.
- It is also the investigator's responsibility to ensure that approval has been granted by both the ethics committee and also the regulatory authority, if applicable (see "The ethics committee" and "Approval from the regulatory authority").
- Once the study has begun, the investigator is responsible for seeing that the protocol is followed, that drugs are distributed and collected correctly, and that the right data is collected. The investigator must also be available for the regular visits that a sponsor makes during the trial (see "Monitoring").
- The investigator is of course always responsible for the patients' safety and that all decisions affecting their treatment be made only by the investigator. The investigator is therefore responsible for keeping informed about developments in the field that the trial covers, and to stay familiarized with any new information concerning any drug being used.
- After the study's completion, the investigator is responsible for ensuring that the patients will continue to receive proper care.

Itemized this way, the duties may seem insurmountable, but in reality many of these responsibilities are already an integrated part of properly functioning health care. Concerning those details that specifically concerns the study, one can often get advice and assistance from a serious sponsor.

The sponsor's responsibility

The sponsor is the partner who initiates, organizes and monitors a clinical trial and/or arranges the financing. Most commonly, it is a pharmaceutical company or a manufacturer of a medical device who is the sponsor, but

16

research foundations, other organizations or even private individuals may also be the sponsors. The text to follow in this chapter mainly describes the responsibilities inherent to companies acting as sponsors of clinical trials.

- The sponsor is responsible that all information about the drug or medical device, its manufacture, packaging and accompanying documentation are correct. The sponsor is also responsible for regularly updating the investigator about new data regarding the drug or medical device being investigated (see "Investigator's Brochure"). It is also the sponsor's responsibility to select investigators for the study and to assure for itself that these are competent and willing to adhere to GCP, etc.
- The investigator and sponsor share mutual responsibility for ensuring that approval for the study has been granted by both ethics committee and the applicable regulatory authority (see "The ethics committee" and "Approval from the regulatory authority"). The sponsor is further obligated for ensuring itself that any permits needed to gain direct access to the patients' medical records are obtained (see "Ensuring the patient's confidentiality").
- The sponsor is required to have a written, documented system (see "SOP") for monitoring and following up clinical trials. This comprises having specially selected and trained persons – clinical monitors – who are the sponsor's representatives and who work closely with the investigators. These have specific duties before, during and after a study (see "The clinical monitor").
- The sponsor is responsible for all drugs involved as concerns their manufacture, packaging, quality and labeling. Routines are required for emergency situations in which the treatment codes for individual patients may need to be broken, and the sponsor is responsible to have someone available around the clock who can answer questions in such situations. The sponsor must also save samples of each drug used in a trial in case there is a later need to perform control analyses. Concerning medical devices the manufacturer is correspondingly responsible for manufacturing, quality, performance, etc.
- Concerning adverse events, the sponsor is responsible for reporting all such to the ethics committee and/or regulatory authority according to a well-defined system (see "Adverse events – side-effects and others").
- The sponsor is responsible for gathering all data from all trials and must also have an internal verification system for monitoring the quality of the trials (see "Audits, inspections and quality assurance").

- Finally, the sponsor, as well as the investigator, is required to archive all documents and collected data. The ICH GCP guidelines describe a relatively intricate procedure in which the required archiving time is based on when the product was registered in the participating ICH countries. This results in the investigator having to hang on to the information until confirmation arrives from the sponsor that it is no longer needed. Concerning data from drug studies, as a result of the international product liability laws, it is also required that the company continues to save much of the study documentation as long as the drug is being sold anywhere in the world, and after that, for an additional number of years. The documents to be stored are those necessary for reconstructing the study afterwards; for example the original data. There is a list in the ICH GCP guidelines covering which documents must be stored.

It is now relatively common that a company out-sources the actual performance of the trial to independent companies know as Contract Research Organizations (CRO's). However, the sponsor retains responsibility for the study even if it is not their own personnel who carries out each stage. All such duties that are contracted out to a CRO must be done so in writing.

It is important to realize that for any study lacking an "outside" sponsor, it is the investigator who assumes all responsibility that would otherwise be the responsibility of the sponsor, such as quality control etc. (see "Monitoring").

SOP – "Standard Operating Procedure"

Companies that carry out clinical trials are required to have an internal, established and written procedure for how these are to be carried out – a Standard Operating Procedure (SOP). This SOP should specify how all parts of a clinical trial are to be performed and monitored from the sponsor's point of view. SOP's should be constructed to satisfy the high standards of Good Clinical Practice and to be a practical handbook for the sponsor's personnel.

A SOP describes both what the company is required to do and what the company requires of the investigator. This should not be viewed as something negative, instead it is a guarantee that the company wants to hold a high standard in its clinical trials. The SOP's are constructed to adhere to GCP and the requirements of various authorities. Because clinical research

18

is an exceptionally international phenomenon, and a SOP is written to be applicable throughout the world, some of the requirements may sometimes seem strange from a local prospective. The areas most often resulting in discussions between sponsor and investigator include the patients' informed consent to participate in the study and the patients' integrity/ secrecy rights (these sections will be discussed in greater detail later in this handbook). In an eagerness to satisfy all conceivable requirements concerning documentation, some companies can go too far in their demands on how things are to be documented etc. Should any requirement seem unreasonably troublesome, the investigator may be wise to verify personally that the requested item is actually specified in the various GCP guidelines – sometimes doing so may result in avoiding administrative routines that makes the study particularly difficult to carry out without contributing any additional quality.

In other words, prior to undertaking a trial it may be wise to ask the sponsor if they have a Standard Operating Procedure – which is required of them – and is there are any specific demands, beyond that of GCP, that these SOP's poses on the investigator and how the trial is to be performed. In actuality, the question should never be necessary, since the sponsor's responsibilities include assuring itself that the investigator is aware of which requirements the GCP and other guidelines place on the performance of the study. During the preparations for the study there ought thus to be many occasions to discuss this with the sponsor.

The "Investigators Brochure"

In clinical trials of drugs or medical devices it is the sponsor's obligation to provide complete information about the drug or device to the participating physicians. This is usually done using an "Investigators Brochure." It should not be older than one year, and is to contain information about the substance's composition and properties, results from animal studies performed for pharmacology, pharmacokinetic and toxicology studies and, depending on how long the drug is supposed to be administered, carcinogenic and teratogenic studies. The results of previous studies in humans must also to be reviewed. It commonly contains a shorter summary of the compound's properties, a description of the reasons behind developing this specific kind of drug and an evaluation of safety aspects. If previous studies have led to suspicions that any particular type of adverse reactions might arise, this should be stated. The ICH GCP guidelines contains relatively detailed instructions about what should be included in an Investigators Brochure.

Concerning medical devices, the contents take another form, naturally. For example, technical performance must be stated as well as which standards the device fulfills. Also required are sections on usage instructions, instructions for installation, maintenance, cleaning etc. If the device has direct contact with the body, or with some other device or drug that itself has direct contact with the body, the material comprising the device and the process of its manufacture must be described in order to be able to determine if there is any risk for unfavorable biological reactions.

An Investigator's Brochure is required also for drugs or devices that are already on the market, although the brochure is often considerably shorter. For example, for a drug it may suffice to simply reproduce the SmPC (Summary of Product Characteristics), Package Insert or similar, plus a summary of the experience and theories that led to consideration of initiating a new test.

It is the investigator's responsibility to read and become familiar with the Investigators Brochure or its equivalent.

It is the sponsor's duty to keep the investigator informed about newly received results, especially those concerning safety aspects, and it is the investigator's duty to keep himself up-to-date with this information. Concerning protracted studies therefor, it is important that the Investigators Brochure or its equivalent be updated at least once yearly. Those Investigators Brochures that were applicable during a study must be archived by the sponsor, and the investigator's documentation (study file) is to contain the most recent revision, along with a list of which other revisions were applicable during the study (see "Documentation and archiving").

The information found in the Investigators Brochures is confidential and may not be disseminated without the sponsor's permission. In general the sponsor probably has no objection to spreading the clinical data about the drug, however the sponsor may want to keep technical data and results such as data from animal studies and pharmacological studies confidential, at least until the drug is registered. There are thus good reasons for the sponsor to desire keeping the clinical information confidential for a given time period, and this is something that must be respected, of course. Before the Investigators Brochure is handed over, the investigator is often requested to sign a special secrecy agreement, in which is stated how the information is to be handled by the investigator. This is often especially emphasized and detailed concerning medical devices.

The clinical trial monitor

The sponsor employs a person who is responsible for the regular contacts with the investigator, and is called the clinical trial monitor, clinical research associate, manager or executive or one of several other titles. This person may have a diverse background, often medical or pharmaceutical training, and is required to have special training for clinical trials, with an education that is suitable to the current study's characteristics. Broadly defined, it is the clinical monitor's job to see to it that the trial is carried out and reported according to the specifications stated in the protocol, while maintaining protection for the patients' integrity and safety.

The clinical monitor has a number of duties before, during and after the study.

Prior to the study, it is the monitor's responsibility to ensure that the investigator and other personnel have the necessary skills. In addition, the monitor must also make sure that the investigator has studied the existing information concerning the drug or equipment, is well-informed about the protocol's content and understands all commitments prior to undertaking the study, such as those concerning GCP, for example. Also included in the information is an evaluation of the available resources – and patients – at the clinic. Procedures for the drug's or device's handling needs to be reviewed, as well as when – and how – the patient code may be broken. The monitor goes through the protocol and the Case Report Form together with the investigator and also ensures that other personnel involved are informed. The monitor also needs to make sure that permits are applied for and received from ethics committees and applicable regulatory authorities.

During the study the clinical monitor must keep in regular contact with the investigator and make regular visits. During these visits they discuss the progress of the study – how many patients have been included, withdrawn, etc. The monitor checks to make sure that the patients' consent has been given before beginning any of the study procedures. In addition, each Case Report Form is reviewed not only to make sure that the protocol is followed, but also to discover any mistakes or overlooked information. This ongoing monitoring considerably improves the possibility of having a correct and complete database at the end of the study. The clinical monitor also performs random tests against the original data; for example, by controlling a given category of information in the original patient charts, and then comparing it with the information in the Case Report Form. The clinical monitor also checks whether the drug or medical device is being properly handled. It is the duty of the clinical monitor to inform the investigator about new data concerning the drug in question. The clinical monitor also regularly checks whether ongoing and required resources are still available, and that all staff concerned are properly informed about the study, etc.

The monitor must document all contact with the investigator, whether this takes place via a visit, written correspondence or telephone conversation. In addition, there must be a list covering the monitor's visits, preferably countersigned by the investigator or other co-worker. Should any significant decision be arrived at during or following the visit, these too must be documented through written correspondence.

After the end of the study, the clinical monitor gathers all Case Report Forms, remaining test drug, code envelopes etc., and verifies that all necessary information is archived in a satisfactory manner by the investigator, and ensures that a report covering the study is written to be sent to the ethics committee and/or applicable authority.

Thus, the investigator and the clinical monitor are going to get well-acquainted with each other. Should the person in question not appear to be suitably compatible, the sponsor can of course always be approached and asked if another monitor could be appointed instead.

The agreement with the sponsor

The agreement between a sponsor and investigator will, of course, vary from case to case depending on the details of each study. Sometimes the study may be entirely initiated by the investigator alone, and the sponsor only contributes with certain financial support, usually in the form of an independent research grant. This does not necessarily require a special written contract, but the sponsor donating the grant usually expects a report about how the research is progressing, most often on a yearly basis, and usually wants a report on any serious adverse events that may occur. It is important to remember that in this type of independent research, it is the investigator who bears the full responsibility for monitoring.

Another situation arises in cases of more conventional clinical trials. The sponsor, usually a pharmaceutical company, a company manufacturing medical devices, or the like, has a vested interest in the results, and accordingly has itself taken the initiative in conducting the study. Even if the investigator's prime motivation for participating in the study should be an interest in the study itself, the work that the investigator and others contribute to the study should, of course, be compensated. The details of this compensation should be careful contracted in writing before the study starts. Even though oral agreements are just as binding as written ones in most legislation, it may be difficult afterwards to prove what was really said should conflict arise. This is specially emphasized in the ICH GCP guidelines, via a statement that such written agreement between the sponsor and the investigator or institution, must exist prior to study start.

Issues that ought to be discussed are the size of the compensation, the applicable rules for its payment, and when it is to be paid.

The size of the compensation can vary enormously depending on the nature of the trial. Long and complicated trials are generally compensated with higher amounts than short and "simple" studies. For investigators and other personnel working as employees of a hospital or institution, there might need to be an agreement concerning how much of the study may be performed during ordinary working hours, and how much has to take place outside these hours. In an increasing number of countries a special contract is required with the responsible employer for the portion taking place during ordinary working hours (see "The contract with the Principal").

In addition to those details that are conducted during ordinary working hours, there is almost always some work that the investigator, and also perhaps even the nurse(s) need to attend to outside of office hours. This can include filling in the Case Report Forms, participating in meetings, etc. Compensation for this work is generally paid directly to the investigator or nurse(s) in various ways. According to local legislation, this may be seen as a spare-time occupation, and each employer may have different provisions concerning this. It may therefor be wise for the prospective investigator to talk with the employer about any possible duty to report such information to the employer.

Another duty for reporting this information has become a hot item of discussion in the last few years; namely whether this compensation must be reported to the ethics committee in connection with the application for conducting a trial. This is currently not the case in most countries, nor do the ICH GCP guidelines so require.

Once there is an agreement on the amount of compensation, there remain several topics to be discussed.

One should, for example, specify the basis on which the compensation is to be calculated. The compensation is normally related to the number of participating patients, and to whether all the patients can be evaluated or not. The study protocol or financial agreement ought to state which patients are evaluable for a prospective analysis, and this can accordingly be used as the basis for calculating the amount of compensation.

Finally, there must be an agreement on *when* the compensation is to be paid. For short studies, it may be entirely adequate that the entire amount be paid at the conclusion of the study. For longer studies, the compensation is usually paid out in increments, and rules for this should be specified. The final payment is generally not paid until all patients are completed, all data collected and the report written.

It has become increasingly common that companies have printed standard contracts covering these aspects. Also included are provisos on what is to take place should the trial not proceed as intended, or if, due to newly available data, the study needs to be changed or canceled altogether. This sort of contract may sometimes feel overly formal, but it provides security to all parties involved should things start falling apart. Even if the contractual wordings may feel unnecessarily bureaucratic at times, this kind of contract is warmly recommended. In many countries it has become mandatory to show these type of contracts to the investigators main employer.

It is not entirely uncommon for the investigator to agree to participate in a clinical study without ever having discussed the economic issues. While this may speak well of the investigator's reasons for participating in the study, it is not at all "suspect" to discuss pecuniary compensation for one's work, and an open discussion "before" can avoid many conflicts "later." The relations between the investigator and the company should be one of mutual respect for each others contributions and roles in developing new drugs, and a professional discussion of monetary matters is definitely a part of this relation.

IND studies

IND refers to "Investigational New Drug" and is a US concept that could be increasingly affecting non-US investigators. When a drug is to be tested in the US, the available pre-clinical and clinical documentation is sent to the FDA as a "IND-application." In the application the company reviews the intended study program for documenting the drug, and broadly describes the various main studies that are planned. The trials that the FDA authorizes via its approval of this application must then be carried out according to US federal law. Especially strict review occurs for drugs that are tested, manufactured and exported abroad directly from the US. That is, these applications will not be approved unless the doctor signing the application commits himself to following the US federal regulations!

Once this decision has been made, a FDA 1572 form will have to be filled in. This document commits the undersigned to follow US federal law on how clinical trials are to be performed. Some of these laws may conflict with local national law and guidelines – the most common conflicts concern full access to original data, composition of ethics committees, some aspects of study monitoring, and the wording of the patient information. It is wise to discuss with the sponsor in advance if this is the case in ones own country and if so, how these matters are to be resolved. It has lately become accepted by the FDA that non US investigators substitute a letter indicating that they will comply with ICH GCP guidelines, however, this should be agreed with the FDA in advance for the study in question.

3 The carrying through

Before

Preparations – visits, planning

Before the investigator and the sponsor reach agreement about starting a clinical trial, the sponsor, often represented by the clinical monitor (see "The clinical monitor"), pays a visit (often several) to the clinic. This is an excellent opportunity to discuss the protocol in more detail, but many other matters will also be discussed.

The sponsor will want to know more about the participating physicians' qualifications and experience with clinical trials or other research projects. Other aspects sponsors are often interested in include:

- are there resources available in the form of time and staff to carry out the project?
- how does the investigator evaluate the proposed methods to be used in the study and are those methods routinely used?
- are there enough patients for inclusion?
- are other projects underway at the center that can hinder the proposed trial?

The investigator in turn ought to take the opportunity to ask questions like:

- How does the sponsor intend to monitor the study once underway? (more on this topic further into the handbook)
- Who will be analyzing the trial's data and how will they be published?
- If applicable, how will the sponsor's economic support be paid – and when?

The first visit(s) are usually spent in wide-ranging discussions about general topics. Once both partners are in agreement that a clinical trial will be started, the sponsor's visits will take on a more practical nature. Agreements are made about how to inform the staff, whether any specific training is required, how the patients' charts are to be recorded, how often the sponsor is to visit, an so on.

These meetings provide the investigator a good opportunity to get to know the sponsor's people who will be working on the study. It also provides an opportunity to evaluate the sponsor's ability and attitude about running clinical trials – a very important issue.

The Study Protocol

The protocol – the trial's overall plan – must contain all the information needed for carrying out the study.

A proposed protocol from the sponsor is often available at an early phase, but since it is the protocol that determines how the study is performed, it is vital that an opportunity exists for discussing the final draft in detail. Both practical and scientific issues should be reviewed. A well-designed protocol is often the foundation of a well-performed study, and the time spent in working through the protocol is time well spent. The protocol discusses not only the main purpose of the study, but also which actions are required to reach this goal. It is not only the purely practical matters that need to be discussed, but also the proposed research methodology itself.

Selected portions of the protocol will be described in detail in a later section of this handbook, but the overall contents will be presented below. It is worth pointing out that is the investigator's duty to become very well acquainted with the protocol.

The title page usually states the study's title, the principal investigator's name, position and telephone number, the other participating investigators' names (with or without address), the sponsor's name, address and telephone number, the sponsor's contact person, and a date that indicates when the protocol was written. Each time the protocol is revised a new date is added for identifying the applicable protocol. It is also a very good idea to date each page in order to avoid confusion among the different revisions. While this may seem obvious, one of the most common problems occurring during checks made by the sponsor or authorities is in identifying which protocol was actually being used (not to mention which one was approved by the ethics committee).

Summary and introduction

The protocol often begins with a summary or synopsis that concisely describes what type of study is intended, the study design, the treatment methods to be used, the dosage (for drugs), and briefly how the study will be carried out.

Following this, an introduction or description of the background factors appears that describes both the reasons for carrying out this specific study and the treatment methods to be used. In drug trials, the new, unknown compound is usually described in some detail. The purpose is to give a background for why the study is being carried out and to state the reasons for why these specific treatment methods were chosen. The general idea is to include sufficient detail to enable a knowledgeable but outside assessor to read this material and then be able to agree that the idea of carrying out this particular study seems sound. This may make it necessary that the section be quite detailed, especially when new drugs or treatment principles are involved. On the other hand this automatically ensures that a good background description has been written, which is needed in any case once the results are to be reported or published, and thus is never wasted effort.

Objectives

The study objectives must be clearly stated. It is generally wise not to address too many research questions at once. Certainly, several objectives can exist, but a single objective should be pointed out as being primary, if for no other reason than to build the basis for statistical calculation of the necessary number of patients to include. The importance of having a well-defined objective cannot be overemphasized. The entire study's design, selection of measurement instruments etc., depends on specifically what is truly intended to study, and it is particularly important that this be made clear from the start. Furthermore, it is also the stated objective that is evaluated by the regulatory agencies and is compared to any possible risks by the ethics committee.

Design

A section about the study design must be included. The most dependable study designs of new compounds are randomized, comparative and double-blind, which means that neither the investigator (and staff) nor patient knows who is receiving which compound. Preferably even the person performing the subsequent statistical analysis shouldn't know until after the analysis (triple blind). An attempt must always be made to keep the investigator's own perceptions of the possible treatment effects from having a chance to affect the results ("bias"). It is virtually impossible to be completely objective when performing a clinical trial – in fact they would probably never be carried out at all if no one believed that one alternative in some manner was better than the other. In order to prevent this from influencing the results, the double-blind study is the golden norm. Should this not be possible for any reason, a detailed explanation is necessary. It is entirely possible to perform a good clinical trial using other designs; however, these will require special caution in order to obtain reliable results. In the case of testing new medical devices, it is often quite impossible to create a blinded study, and therefore the possibility of having the data analyzed in a blind fashion – i.e., a third party etc. – should be specially considered.

The patient population

The section about the patient population principally discusses the issues of how many patients are required and which ones should be included in the study.

How many is primarily determined by statistical calculation and in a few cases by practical limitations in patient availability. The section that discusses calculations of sample size (the number of patients to be included) ought to be rather detailed. All international guidelines stress the importance of a thorough calculation of sample size. The required number of patients to be included is based on: the expected drug effects, their variability, the amount of difference needed between the two treatment regimes to claim clinical significance, and the desired statistical power to support this claim. At times it is impossible to know exactly what effects can be expected, although it is often possible to estimate on the basis of data from other, similar drugs. Should this not be possible either, then an explanation for this should be given in the protocol.

Which patients to study is specified using inclusion and exclusion criteria. The inclusion criteria are generally relatively few in number and describe the general patient population under consideration for the study. They are thus generally broad in nature – for example, men and women between the ages of 18 and 70, and who are afflicted by the disease under study, according to some standard norm. The exclusion criteria, however, are generally numerous and describe all exceptions from the general rule. They aim, in part, to screen out those patients who should be excluded due to reasons of safety like pregnant or nursing women. They are also used to achieve a somewhat more homogenous group of patients who do not have too many confounding factors; that is, factors that can affect or disturb the results in any manner. The optimal balance between inclusion and exclusion is not always easy to determine. For example, having few exclusion criteria make it considerably easier to collect a sufficient patient population within a reasonable amount of time; on the other hand, the patient group will then be less homogenous and the corresponding results can therefore become much less conclusive. On yet a third hand, a more heterogeneous patient group may better resemble the total patient population and the results, once obtained, may therefore be more generally applicable.

Some types of trials may require a specially selected patient sample, or that patients do – or refrain from doing – certain things. Such considerations must be carefully described. Certain inherent characteristics of the selected patients may affect the treatment method's efficacy, and thus a detailed description is needed about how an even distribution of these characteristics will be achieved in the different study groups (stratified randomization).

Practical execution

The protocol is also to describe the practical execution of the study, visit by visit. Here should be explained what needs to be done at different occasions, the times between visits, the maximum allowable deviations from these intervals, and so on. At an early stage careful consideration should be paid to whether it is truly possible to follow the study plan. For example, is the clinic closed for vacations during a period that patients should be receiving a treatment? Are the treatments planned for a part of the day that could conflict with other activities?

There should also be a flowchart that briefly but clearly lists the actions to be done at each visit. If the protocol is written in English, which is usually the case, it can be a good idea to translate the flowchart to the national language(s). This allows it to be used by the staff as an easily comprehended guide. The protocol should also state which treatment the patients are to receive following the study's conclusion. This can be specially sensitive in trials studying drugs or devices in an early phase of development and intended for use in a serious disease where no effective treatment currently exists. A very difficult ethical problem can arise when the study ends and thus the question of whether to terminate a possibly functioning treatment while on the other hand there still isn't sufficient documentation to demonstrate that the drug is safe and efficacious in the long run. This needs to be thoroughly discussed in advance and described in the protocol so that the ethics committee has a chance to evaluate the problem and the patients can be properly informed.

There must be both a specification of and reasons stated for the choice of treatment; and concerning drugs, justifications of the dosage, dose interval and time of day for taking the drug are also necessary. It is important that the drugs in comparable studies are used at approximately equipotent doses; that is, that the study is a comparison of different drugs at clinically comparable dosages. Likewise it is important that the treatment method being tested against is a currently accepted one. The ethical aspects of a placebo-controlled study should be especially considered. Very often placebo treatment for short time periods present no problems; it is when the treatments begin to approach longer time periods, or in emergency situations, that problems can arise. The permissibility of additional medication during the study should also be stated, as well as how one is to proceed with patients who require dose adjustments for one reason or another. It is also necessary to describe how one is to evaluate patient compliance.

Timetable

The protocol should also include a study timetable stating the preliminary date that the final report is expected.

Composition and handling of experimental compounds

A description of the experimental drug's composition is required; for example whether capsules or tablets will be used, or whether the compounds resemble each other etc. Packaging size, dosing instructions and labeling should also be stated. The labeling must clearly state that the drugs are intended only for use in clinical trials. The clinical trial must be identifiable, usually using a study number, and both the investigator and the manufacturer must be identified. The drug must be marked (for example, ABC 123/placebo) as well as the amount, dosage and mode of administration. Instructions for storage, including a statement about keeping the compound out of reach of children, is also required. Double-blind studies require that each patient have a specially packaged drug labeled with the patient number or its equivalent. An expiration date for the drug must also be included. It is important that this labeling be done in such manner that it is impossible to see the difference between the two drugs. The labeling must normally be written in the national language(s). One possible exception to this is using English labeling for substances that are never handled by any other person than the investigator, such as radio labeled, directly administered substances. Drugs intended for clinical testing may not be administered to other patients; and this is usually stated in the protocol.

Another question that needs to be discussed concerning the drug itself, is how it is to be handled. A careful accounting is required of which substance has been given to which patient, as well as when and what the patients return. In principle, it must be possible to precisely account for where each table has gone, and the various tallies must agree. After the end of the study, the drug should then be destroyed and the destruction documented; this is normally done by the sponsor, but the pharmacy can sometimes be of assistance with this.

Use of medical devices

The national language(s) should be used in instructions for usage, maintenance, and cleaning of medical devices, the contents of these instructions must also be described, and a description included about how these are to be distributed to the staff and patients. The protocol must also state whether a cooperative contact will be made with the hospital's medical technology section.

The device should be clearly labeled that it is intended only for use in clinical trials, its identity (designation, manufacturing number, batch number, date of manufacture etc.) and the manufacture's and investigator's names and addresses. This labeling should use the national language(s).

The sponsors continuing commitments

Another practical detail that should be stated in the protocol is how the sponsor will honor its commitments concerning its control measures during the study. These include, for example, regular visits (see "Monitoring"), following up information provided to the staff, any quality controls (see "Audits, inspections and quality assurance") and so on. In some of the cases, such as when the sponsor merely contributes economic support or free substances without having a direct interest the study itself, the sponsor will not provide these functions, and this should clearly be stated in the protocol. In these cases, it is the investigator alone who is the guarantor that the study is carried out properly, including the responsibility to monitor the study. Should this arrangement be a multi-center study with many participants, it becomes a heavy responsibility to be assumed by the investigator.

Randomization

Randomization procedures are an essential aspect – errors made here can invalidate the results – and thus these must be described in detail. Both the time at which the randomization is to occur and whether it is stratified must be stated. Stratification can become necessary in studies where inherent factors present in the population may be expected to have prognostic significance for the outcome (confounding factors). One such example is the knowledge that smokers and nonsmokers react differently to a given treatment. In this case it is necessary to try to achieve an even distribution of smokers and nonsmokers in the various treatment groups being studied; and especially concerning smaller studies, it may therefor be necessary to stratify the actual randomization. Stratification can significantly complicate the randomization procedure if more than one or two factors are to be weighed in. However, the techniques in this field have advanced considerably in recent years, and today there are good possibilities of conducting a stratified randomization where a large number of factors can be considered. This is done using computer programs that can be programmed for a large number of factors. However, this assumes that the randomization is done centrally at one location; it can also cause several practical complications concerning how the blinding is to be maintained, how to ensure that the patients receive the correct treatment, etc. Thus, the choice of a stratified randomization must be well-justified and thought through in respect to the practical consequences.

Breaking the treatment codes

Another required section is instructions on who is allowed to break the treatment codes for a patient, under which circumstances and how this is actually to be done. Randomized, double-blind studies commonly use a list of randomization codes for all patients and one envelope per patient with an individualized code. These envelopes are usually retained in duplicate, with one copy for the investigator, and the other(s) for the pharmacy, safety committee, or sponsor. This ensures that there always is a possibility of breaking the code in case of emergency with any given patient.

Breaking the code (for example, for an interim analyses for an entire study) may be necessary at times for reasons of both efficacy and safety. Interim analyses should preferably not be attempted while the study is in progress, but at times it is a necessary evil brought about by safety reasons (to name but one). There are accepted, but complicated, techniques for these kinds of interim analysis. Should interim analyses be planned for, the reasons for doing so must be thoroughly and well justified. Interim analyses can also be conducted without breaking the code – it is enough to distinguish group A from group B, and it is not necessary to know which group is which in order to perform the analysis.

Withdrawals

A separate section should exist that discusses patients who withdraw from the study for whatever reason. There may be special procedures to be performed in case of withdrawals and there may also be circumstances where the patient's data may still be "usable" to the study in certain aspects. All patients included in the study must be reviewed afterwards, and even if withdrawn may still be included in certain analyses depending on the reason for withdrawing. When the number of required patients for the study is calculated, a certain drop-out rate ought to be expected and planned for in the early planning stages of the study in order to secure a sufficient number of evaluable patients.

Evaluation of efficacy

Methods included in the study, such as those used for the evaluation of efficacy and safety, must be described. This is especially important for multicenter trials, i.e., those with more than one participating center. For the study to be reliable, the efficacy must be measured with the same techniques at all centers. At times this could require the use of rather complicated standardization methods to guarantee this. It has become increasingly common that the efficacy variable is evaluated by a central unit even when the data has been gathered elsewhere, for example, that all ECG's be evaluated at one center, or that all blood samples are analyzed by a single laboratory; however, this is not always possible. Should central evaluation not be possible, it is necessary for the various investigators to have the possibility of meeting regularly throughout the study in order to maintain coordination at this level. The protocol must also state how the efficacy variable is to be evaluated and what requirements are necessary in order to classify the patients' response to treatment, etc. This is especially important if the efficacy variable is subject to subjective evaluation, such as an estimate on a descriptive scale. These type of variables may necessitate repeated trial runs in which the participating investigators practice making reproducible and consistent evaluations, and get a chance to discuss differences in their evaluations.

This is extra important in studies in which, for whatever reason, the treatments are given openly. One common method is to use an independent "end-point committee," which is a group of specialists who have no other contact with the study, and who can evaluate the efficacy "blindly"; that is, without knowing which treatment any particular patient has received. One type of such technique that has come into use in large mortality studies is the PROBE design, which stands for Prospective, Randomized, Open, Blinded Evaluation. The patients are openly treated, often using regularly prescribed drugs, but the evaluation of all "end-points," that is the primary efficacy variables, are made by an independent committee who receives all its materials "blinded," meaning that all information that identifies which drug treatment the patient has received has been omitted. This or similar kinds of studies naturally require much consideration in order to work properly, but may be the only option for carrying out very large and long studies. Another variation of large mega-studies are the large cardiovascular studies run on an international basis, such as the ISIS studies. These studies are run using blinded drugs and sometimes placebo, but the actual study conduct and data collection have been simplified in the extreme. No true monitoring in the form of site visits has been done. The ICH GCP guidelines have seized upon this kind of study design as being both important and possible, and states that a specific exemption from the monitoring requirement at each study site may be acceptable for certain types of studies, in which case this must be motivated and described in the protocol.

Statistics

The statistical aspects require their own, thoroughly described section that discusses the basis for the sample size (which often entails an estimate of the expected efficacy and its variability) and an estimate of which differences can be valuable to discover. Sometimes it is simply impossible to exactly predict the size of the expected efficacy and a more general reasoning must suffice.

In this section, a description of how the study results are to be analyzed must be stated. If possible, this section should cover the choice of the intended statistical methods, their levels of significance, and how much statistical power is desired.

Also needed is a definition of which patients will be included in the analyses, the "intention-to-treat" (namely, all patients randomized into the study) or "on-treatment" (meaning all patients who correctly completed the study, also often called the "per-protocol analysis"). Subgroup analyses may also occur, which is sometimes important for the calculation of the total number of required patients. The use of subgroup analyses should be clearly stated before the trial begins.

As discussed above, some kinds of studies may require interim analyses – usually for safety reasons. Because the performance of such analyses can affect the statistical calculations for the study in its entirety, it is wise to seek out professional help in order to perform these analyses correctly, not only concerning how to do an interim analysis, but also for estimating the effect they will have on the final analyses.

Because the various statistical calculations are the foundation for designing the entire study and can have far-reaching consequences for the number of patients, the potential for carrying out the study and so forth, the importance of a sound statistical description cannot be pointed out too often. Unfortunately, the statistical foundations in many studies are rather meager, something that many a investigator has bitterly regretted – afterwards …

Safety and ethical aspects

All clinical trials, indeed all human experimental research, must be approved by an ethics committee, and if it concerns the testing of experimental compounds, often also by the local regulatory authorities (see "Approval from the regulatory agency"). Since this is regulated by guidelines and local regulations it is not always specified in the protocol that an application is to be made. However, there needs to be a section in the protocol about the ethical aspects of the research, and each investigator must reach an individual decision that the possible benefits outweigh the possible risks, and that risk is minimized. Written information for the patient is obligatory and must be appended to the protocol. Also required is a description of how information to the participants is to be presented, and how their consent is to be obtained. In addition, in many countries it is also required to submit a copy of any advertisement concerning patient recruitment. Careful instructions concerning how adverse events are to be reported must be included, including a time frame specifying the nature of the adverse event and its severity (see "Adverse events – side-effects and others"). The ethical principles that governs all clinical research are described in the Helsinki Declaration, which is often appended to the protocol, and is included in this handbook (Appendix 1). Ethical aspects are treated in more detail in the section entitled "Ethical considerations".

There is another safety aspect than those purely related to adverse reactions. This concerns the carrying out of the study and the test results. In intervention studies, especially those intended to reduce mortality for a given disease, the test results obtained during the study may make it unethical to continue. It may turn out that the new therapy does not have a sufficient efficacy or – which results in the same ethical problem – the new therapy leads to a much improved efficacy. In either case it is unethical to continue treating the patients with the inferior alternative. In order to discover this, it is necessary to build into the study a checkpoint along the way, in which the result up to that point can be analyzed (interim analyses). This is possible, although rather complicated from a statistical point of view; and it ought to be carefully discussed in advance how this is to be done and who decides when to break off the study. From a methodological viewpoint interim analyses should always be avoided, and it is only in certain kinds of studies that they should even be considered – such as a therapy for an previously untreatable and severe illness. Very often an independent safety committee is established for this purpose, whose only function is to control the safety aspects, but is otherwise uninvolved in the study.

This committee is to monitor the study by adhering to a previously drawn up program, and the committee's members are the only ones who have access to these results while the trial is running. Often this can be done blindly, that is the committee only gets access to data recorded as group A or B, without knowing which group has received which treatment. Only when the difference between the two groups becomes too large to allow the study to continue are the codes broken for the two groups. In order to make the correct decision, it is generally necessary to include statistical expertise in the committee alongside the medical. However, when evaluating treatment of severely ill patients with a complex clinical profile it is often necessary for the committee to evaluate the data un-blinded, in order to be able to discern a pattern of increasing side effects, aggravated disease etc.

Information/delegation to the staff

The ICH GCP guidelines also emphasizes the relationship between the investigator and other staff involved and the necessity to decide who does what, and document this, before the start of the study. This can be done in the protocol, but perhaps more easily in a separate delegation and signature list.

Other points that might need to be specified in the protocol are sections about insurance for – and possible compensation to – patients, a description of how the results are to be published, and how the archiving of trial documentation is to occur.

A vast number of other details, depending on the type of study, can also be included in the protocol. Because the protocol is the study's "bible," many practical details may be included. This often makes the protocol rather bulky, which is something that simply must be quietly put up with. Once the study is underway, a simplified flowchart is usually sufficient, and the protocol then serves as a reference source.

The Case Report Form

The Case Report Form (Case Report – or Record – Form, called the "CRF") is the document into which all the data necessary for analysis is to be recorded. The form's design may vary, but it often take the shape of one notebook per patient – and is often more extensive than expected. All essential information is recorded in these notebooks, patient by patient and visit by visit. It is advantageous if each section in the notebook is accompanied by instructions concerning what should be recorded at every specific occasion. While this information may be found in the study protocol, it considerably facilitates practical operations to repeat the instructions in the CRF. Once the study is underway it is the CRF that is in daily use, and it is practical and convenient not to have to refer to the study protocol during each visit.

The CRF is often designed to facilitate data analysis. At times this makes them somewhat clumsy from the clinician's point of view. Unreasonably impractical CRFs should not be accepted, since they endanger a smooth and consistent data collection. It does not help much if a CRF is very easy to enter into a computer database, if its construction has made it almost impossible to complete in the first place.

Naturally, the actual appearance of the form will vary considerably from study to study and from sponsor to sponsor. A more compact form with much information to be reported on each page may seem attractive due to its lesser bulk. However a more "sparse" form requiring less data per page may be easier to fill in, despite any initial shock on seeing its thickness for the first time.

The data in the CRF is to be filled in by the investigator or any person formally delegated to carry out the procedure in question. Those receiving authorization to fill in the data in the CRF – and preferably a specification of which data it applies to – must be documented on a special "signature-list," which is to be updated as needed during the study and archived afterwards (see "Study documentation). It is ultimately the investigator who accepts responsibility for the correctness of these data via his or her signature.

If for some reason the data needs to be revised in the CRF, the old data should be crossed over, not erased, and the revision is to be dated and initialed. In addition a reason for the revision needs to be stated if it isn't immediately obvious in context.

The data that is recorded in the CRF also needs to be entered into the patient's regular chart, which is the source document. All pertinent data must be recorded in the patient chart in case it is needed in the future for data verification (see sections: "Monitoring," "Audits" and "Documentation and archiving"). However, in some cases some of the original data collected for the study can be of such nature that they are not very suitable for archiving in the patient's regular chart. For example, this may occur if a large number of extra examinations are conducted exclusively for reasons related to the study, and lack significance for the patient's continued care. There is a not insignificant risk that much of such data will later be excised from the chart. It is then better to archive them in, or along with, the CRF. When this procedure is chosen it should be stated in the patient's chart from the study start. This is also true concerning other data documented directly into the CRF, such as replies to specific questionnaires or forms. The location where the data is first documented is, of course, original data – in this case the CRF itself. This is entirely acceptable, but requires description in the patient chart at the start of the study, so that one can always know where to find the original information. According to the ICH GCP guidelines a statement must be added to the protocol that this method (i.e. using the CRF as source data for some variables) has been chosen and which data it applies to.

Ethical considerations

The relationship between doctors and their patients during research were first widely disseminated in writing in 1947 as the Nuremberg Code. This was later further developed as the Helsinki Declaration and was adopted in 1964, and later revised in 1975, 1983, 1989 and 1996 and is under continuous revision. This document maintains that a doctor's first responsibility is always to protect the people's health. It also ascertains that the development of new, effective treatment methods unavoidably involve experimentation using humans, experiments that can be potentially risky. What must then be complied with in order that such experiments, such as clinical trials, can be carried out?

First and foremost, established scientific methodology must be used. The experiment must be substantiated using laboratory data and animal data as much as possible, and investigators are required to be extensively read in the relevant literature.

A carefully constructed protocol must be written and submitted to an independent group for evaluation (an ethics committee).

The person running the test must be scientifically qualified and the risk to the individual participating patients must not exceed the expected beneficial results neither for the patient himself/herself nor for a larger group of patients. It also emphasizes that the research subject's integrity is to be protected at all times, that the participation must be voluntary and consented to only after being accurately informed about every aspect of the experiment.

In addition, when the study subjects are also the doctor's own patients, it becomes especially important that the patient's dependence is not exploited, and that it is perfectly clear that a refusal to participate will not in any manner affect the patient's own treatment. A respect for the patient's best interest must always be kept in mind and the doctor is always responsible for the patient receiving the best possible treatment at every given occasion. It is also stated that the researcher is responsible for the correctness of the findings in publication, and that any study not adhering to these ethical rules not be accepted for publication.

What does this mean in purely practical terms with respect to clinical trials?

The gist of the matter is that every physician is free to participate in clinical trials, but he/she must be convinced that the project is ethically defensible. There are a great many factors that must be evaluated.

Can the study's findings be of use to the participating patient – or perhaps a larger group of patients? Is the studied designed using sound scientific methodology? Are the chosen methods sufficiently evaluated and the study designed in a manner that will truly lead to conclusive results? It may seem obvious that such must be the case, but unfortunately it isn't always so. Deficiencies in the study design (such as too small sample sizes), deficiencies in randomization, efficacy variables that are dependent on each other etc. can make a study completely worthless. To carry out a study that cannot produce evaluable results must be considered unethical, even if the patients are not exposed to risk or discomfort.

In studies that also expose patients to risk or discomfort, as occurs in for example invasive investigations, the requirements must be set even higher. In this case the results must truly benefit the individual patient or a larger group of patients.

It is also necessary to ponder the requirement that the patient must always be given the best possible treatment. If the two intended therapies seem very comparable, or if one of them might conceivably be better, then there is not much of a problem, given that the study is constructed in such a way as to safe guard the patient should the assumptions prove to be untrue. Placebo treatment is another matter. Sometimes there is no available treatment and then placebo treatment is totally acceptable or even preferable, at least until it becomes obvious that the new treatment offers clear advantages. When this happens it is no longer ethically acceptable to continue the placebo treatment, and the study may be discontinued so that all of the patients may be given the new treatment. Another situation arises when there is an alternative treatment, but it still is necessary to compare a new drug with a placebo in order to establish its efficacy, as is often demanded by regulatory authorities. It then becomes necessary for the investigator to be convinced that the patient is not exposed to risk by being treated with placebo, and this often sets a limit to the study's length. That placebo treatment is not automatically unethical has been made clear in the most recent amendment of the Helsinki Declaration (Section II, paragraph 2).

If all of these ethical considerations seem insurmountable, it is sometimes useful to remember that one of a doctor's responsibilities, as expressed by the selfsame declaration, is to gain and maintain knowledge and a high standard of health care for the patient, and one of the best ways to accomplish this is to actively participate in research, such as clinical trials, for example.

The ethics committee

All clinical research projects must be examined and approved by an independent ethics committee (or review board), regardless of whether the drug is already registered or not and regardless of whether patients or healthy volunteers are involved. The investigator is responsible for informing and dealing with the ethics committee as well as being responsible for the patients' welfare. However, the sponsor often assists with the practical management. The application normally needs to be written on a special form that can be obtained from the committee (in some countries national forms exist, in others each committee uses their own format). A copy of the protocol and a copy of the Investigators Brochure or its equivalent are to be appended to the application, and in some countries also the investigator's Curriculum Vitae.

The ethics committee's principal duty is to safeguard the patients' or test subjects' interest (see "Ethical considerations"). Even though it primarily evaluates the ethical aspects of the planned study, it also studies the scientific content. That is, it is not considered ethically defensible to expose people to clinical trials that, due to their design – or more accurately, deficiency in design – cannot lead to any results, even if the patients are not subjected to any risk or discomfort. In those countries where the regulatory authorities are involved, which is becoming the norm in one form or another, it usually remains the regulatory authorities' primary task to examine the scientific design in detail.

Ethics committees base their work on the Helsinki Declaration first written in 1964 (most recently revised in 1996) and committees must include both laymen and experts. The committees must follow a written directive – a SOP if you will – a copy of which should be obtainable from each committee.

The committee judges, among other aspects:

- The study's scientific tenability.
- The investigator's suitability (which requires a certain local knowledge) and prospects for performing the study.
- Whether the risks that the patients are being subjected to have been minimized and are proportional to the study result's expected advantages.
- Whether the patients are correctly selected and informed about the study.

The issue of insurance for the patients, should any untoward effects occur, has become an increasingly important aspect. In some countries, notably some of the Nordic ones, general insurance exists, also covering patients and healthy subjects in clinical trials. In most other countries the individual company insurance carry the bulk of patient coverage in trials. The ethics committee generally requests information about, or confirmation that, such insurance exists,

In addition, the ethics committee generally requests information about how participants are to be economically compensated for their participation in order to evaluate whether the amount is large enough to endanger the assumption of free choice.

Any amendment to the protocol significantly affecting the study or its participants must be submitted to the ethics committee. This can include the need for additional patients, additional laboratory testing etc. Since such changes are of a nature that could alter the committee's prior approval, amendments must be submitted and renewed approval received. Here too, amendments in administrative details are of lesser significance. Because the piling up of administrative changes has a tendency to grow steadily, the workload on the ethics committee members around the world has increased in recent years. Quite often these kinds of changes are of no interest to the ethics committee, and only confer an increased workload and thereby pro-long processing time without providing any improved quality. It may there-for be wise to contact the ethics committee in advance to submitting such routine information. Even the ICH GCP guidelines discuss whether admin-istrative changes must necessarily be approved by the ethics committee. In case of doubt about whether an amendment is of pure administrative nature or not, a simple preliminary contact with the ethics committee may often resolve the matter.

The ethics committee must produce a written decision that also states which persons participated in the decision. It is especially important that there is no prior conflict of interest for anyone assisting in the decision. Since those who are active researchers also tend to be those sitting on research ethics committees, it is not uncommon that someone participating in the research is also sitting on the committee. It is very important that this person does not participate in the decision, and that it is clearly stated so in the list of participants, or in the committee's own minutes from the meeting.

Research ethics committees is one topic that can lead to conflict between US, European and other regulations. US federal regulations contain very detailed instructions on how an ethics committee is to be composed and how it is to proceed. Even though most countries in principle fulfill the majority of these US federal requirements, there remain points that are not in exact agreement. For example, the US federal regulations include descriptions on precisely how many laymen and experts are to sit, their ethnic origins, judicial qualifications, and so forth. This is not always defined in such detail in other countries.

In the US and many other countries, and also in accordance with the ICH GCP guidelines, the ethics committees also have a watchdog role over the study while it is in progress. Both adverse effects and study results etc. are to be reported to the committee.

Patient information and informed consent

One point that ethics committees study particularly carefully is how the patients are informed about the study and how they grant their consent to participate. Many times the patients have a psychologically dependent relationship with the investigator, and thus it is of prime importance that the information about the study is presented well and that the voluntary aspect is very clear. Information for the patient must be presented both verbally and in writing, and must contain at least the following:

- What the study is about and why it is being performed.
- What kind of drugs will be used.
- What methods will be used, why, and whether they are experimental or not.
- The potential for possible discomfort.
- Procedures outside the normal hospital routines.
- Whether a placebo will be used.
- How the study will be carried out.
- Whether alternative treatments exist and what they are.
- That participation is entirely voluntary and that the patient may at any time withdraw from the study without having to explain why; and that doing so will not jeopardize their receiving further optimal treatment.
- That all information gathered in the study will be treated confidentially (and, if so be, computer analyzed) and that it will be impossible for anyone to trace any given person in the final results.
- Possible economic compensation (generally only valid for healthy volunteers or their equivalents. Patients can sometimes be compensated for costs like transportation, cost of other medications, cost for child care so patients can make the study visits, etc., but not payment for participation as such).
- Which persons/physicians bear responsibility for the trial and how to reach them.

The guidelines especially emphasize that the information provided must be understandable to laymen, and it is also important that it isn't so lengthy and detailed that the most important sections get lost in a mass of what could be considered as less essential information.

That information has been presented, *when* this was done and *by whom* must be documented. The protocol must also describe the means by which this is to be done.

After having received the information and been given time to think it through, the patient must grant consent in order to participate ("informed consent"). According to the ICH GCP guidelines the patient must confirm in writing that he/she has been informed about the study and that he/she consents to participation. This form of written consent is not generally something that the patients react negatively to, although there certainly are cultural differences in how the information should be worded and delivered. Anything other than written consent has to be carefully explained, justified and described in the protocol. The protocol must clearly state which procedure is to be used and document that each patient has gone through the entire procedure, prior to the entering the study or any related procedure. Concerning studies on healthy volunteers (described as "non-therapeutic" research in the Helsinki declaration), written consent is mandatory.

A special case arises when patients are not capable of granting informed consent, such as unconscious patients. If the ethics committee decides that it may still be in the patient's best interest, even this group of patients may be studied. In such cases it is the patient's next of kin (or guardian, if one has been appointed) whom is asked instead, and who may grant informed consent. Should the patient later improve to the degree that his/her informed consent is possible, the question may then be put to the patient. Concerning clinical trials on children, it is the child's parent [or guardian] who must grant informed, written consent. Should the child be old enough to understand the issues involved, then the question is put to him/her; and should the child say "no" then his/her wish is to be accepted, even if the parent or guardian said "yes." In Europe the age limit is often put at around 12 to 14 years, but of course this must be adjusted to the child's own degree of mental development. This is also an area were different countries have differing customs which might need to be taken into consideration.

In studies performed according to US standards (see "IND-studies"), the proposed information for the patients can be enormously detailed, and include content that other national ethics committees do not willingly accept. This ought to be discussed with the sponsor on a case-to-case basis, and as a rule, these problems are generally resolvable.

Naturally, providing careful information to patients consumes a considerable amount of time. Besides being the investigator's responsibility to provide comprehensive information, it is in fact time well spent. A patient who has received information about the study in peace and quiet, and has decided to participate, most often becomes a committed and cooperative participant.

Approval from the regulatory authority

In an increasing number of countries, but not all, clinical trials with drugs, experimental compounds (including radio-labeled drugs, herbal remedies and some externally-applied drugs), or medical devices on patients or healthy volunteers, needs to be approved by the pertinent regulatory authority. The form of this application can vary substantially from the US were approval can be sought for an entire development program (see IND applications) to countries like Sweden were each individual trial needs an approval from the regulatory authorities. When the new EU directives are enforced the procedure will become more similar in the different member states, but until that time one had better ascertain the rules applicable to ones own country. The legislation outside the three ICH territories – i.e. US, EU and Japan, can be even more varying – the only general advice can be not to forget to check whether a regulatory approval is needed in addition to the ethical one.

The time needed for approval also varies considerably, from around 4 to 6 weeks up to a year or more!

Although legislation and procedure vary, something can be learned from the problems commonly encountered in those countries were individual trial approval is needed. The most common problems requiring complementary information are:

- poor background for the study and choice of design
- insufficient discussion concerning the dosage chosen
- irrelevant choice of inclusion and exclusion criteria
- irrelevant choice of or inadequate evaluation of endpoints – i.e. the study's efficacy variable(s)
- the statistical foundation for sample size or evaluation

- intended treatment once the study is concluded
- overall Safety Assessment – an evaluation from the investigator or sponsor about the drug's general safety profile and its implications for the study and the patients.

Regulatory authorities can, and do, reject the application to proceed with a clinical study. This is often attributable to the following causes:

- significant weaknesses in the documentation of the drug
- poor pharmaceutical quality of the drug
- toxic effects that can lead to safety risks
- serious deficiencies in the study design that would render the study unevaluable or inconclusive

It sometimes happens, if rarely, that regulatory agencies discontinue an ongoing trial. This may happen when serious risks or unacceptable adverse events appear during the course of the trial, or when significant deviation from the original protocol takes place.

It is not uncommon that a protocol needs to be amended in some manner. This can happen both before and after the start of the study. Especially in the latter case, the changes can be very delicate methodologically, and shouldn't be undertaken unnecessarily, but may be necessary for reasons of safety; for example. Amendments that concern patient safety and/or the possibility of evaluating the study may need to be submitted to the pertinent regulatory authority (and always to the Ethical committee) even when the protocol has already been approved; and in these cases the study may not continue until the new approval has been received.

Some regulatory authorities also want reports about how the study went afterwards. Likewise, should a study not actually take place, the investigator needs to communicate the reasons for this to the regulatory authority in some countries. In some countries studies who go on for longer periods (more than one year) needs to be reported in short to the authorities on a yearly basis. Many authorities also require a final report once the study is concluded. A final report needs to be more extensive, except perhaps when the study was discontinued. In this case the reasons for the discontinuation need to be described in detail. It is assumed that the final report will eventually be published (as an article) or made generally known in some other manner.

Approval from the radiation protection committee or similar

In many countries, but not all, special considerations are necessary when conducting studies with radioactive substances. This mostly arises in Phase I studies when the drug's metabolism in the body is to be studied, but an increasing number of techniques are being developed that use radio-labeled substances in various circumstances. In such cases several countries require that the study be approved by a radiation protection committee or similar, in addition to the usual ethics committees and possible regulatory authorities.

Protecting the patient's confidentiality

Patients participating in clinical trials are covered by the same confidentiality regulations as apply to all patients. This legislation differs around the world, but often includes that only those professional care givers who need this information in order to provide care at the clinic are allowed access to the patient's medical charts. Identifying information about the patient must not be released to others – and this includes clinical monitors – even if these others are registered nursed or physicians in their own right. The information in the CRF must therefore be recorded anonymously such that the patient is only identified with a patient number and initials. Nonetheless, the sponsor must also be able to compare the information in the patient's case report form with the data recorded in the patient's medical charts which can thus be conceived as somewhat of a conflict of interests.

The current guidelines and regulations assume that direct verification will occur. This normally means that permission must be granted from each participating subject – and also that any subject not willing to grant this is not permitted to participate in the clinical trial. Thus a confidentiality agreement is needed in which the patient consents to allowing persons representing the pharmaceutical firm or foreign registration authorities (for example) to have access to their charts during the course of the study. In many countries the wording of such an agreement must be appended to the application to the ethics committee, and is normally limited to being valid only during the time that the study is being run. This type of confidentiality agreement is becoming increasingly common, and most patients do not perceive this as negative, especially if they have had explained to them that the reason is the wish to ensure both ethical and scientific propriety.

In some countries the monitor will also need a permission from the institution or person bearing chief responsibility for maintaining confidentiality, usually the head of clinic or its equivalent. In this agreement, the company's representative pledges in turn to adhere to the regulations on professional secrecy etc.

Information for the staff

Another important informational aspect is how the staff is to be informed, both those directly concerned with performing the trial and other staff that may be expected to come into contact with the patients.

Those directly involved in the trial are usually clinical, laboratory and perhaps department staff. It is the investigator's responsibility to see to it that these staff members are not only informed that a clinical trial is to be performed, but also what the study is about and any special requirements that may occur in different situations. Sometimes the protocol has a special section describing how this is to take place, and specifies what information is supposed to be covered; in additional all the actual provision of information is to be documented.

This is primarily an issue of safety – the desire is to minimize the risk of exposing the patient to unnecessary risks. For example, it may happen that the drugs be to used in the study should not be combined with certain other medications. Another very important aspect with staff information is that it increases the chances that the trial will be performed well and correctly. The investigator naturally cannot always be present and if all the staff has a good understanding of the main purpose of the study many unnecessary mistakes can be avoided.

Two categories of staff who are often overlooked in this connection are laboratory and pharmacy staff. In many trials the various lab findings are a crucial part of the analysis, concerning both efficacy and safety, and it should be obvious that some effort should be made to keep the various lab findings as complete as possible. Nonetheless, it happens that the lab staff remains totally in the dark that a clinical trial is being performed and thus no one there is paying extra attention that specifically these patients tests must be performed correctly and diligently. It may also be a good idea to consult with the lab about working out a means of specially labeling the samples that belong to the trial in order to increase the chances for complete lab data. In some cases the pharmacy is involved in the trial by assisting in the distribution of drugs. Even when the (hospital) pharmacy is not actively involved, it is still worthwhile informing the pharmacy that patients are likely to visit that a clinical trial is underway. Patients often go to the pharmacist with questions about the nature of the medicine they take, and if the pharmacy staff has a basic knowledge about the drug being tested in the trial, they may then assist in avoiding potentially harmful combinations with drugs prescribed by other physicians. This information may take the form of a brief summary sent to the pharmacy, although preferably delivered personally by visiting the pharmacy.

It is the investigator's responsibility to see to it that all relevant staff are informed – and stay informed! Of course, this may require a lot of effort, especially if it is a long-term study and new staff requiring information enter the project. Here is where the sponsor can provide good service, such as having the clinical monitor step in and provide this information. Please note that any disseminated information must be documented as to when and how delivered.

It is wise to remember that the staff is often employed in positions that do not necessarily cover research programs. If the staff is not informed – and turned on to the project – they may instead feel that the trial is no more than an extra burden stealing time from their "real" job. The information surrounding the project thus becomes very important. A pleasant side effect that often occurs is that a well-informed staff feels involved in, and motivated about, the clinic's work and often feels proud and happy about working in a clinic performing research.

The contract with the Principal

Most trials take place in hospitals, institutions or clinics run by someone else than the investigator. This can be government, county councils, universities, private enterprises and so forth. Quite often the financial agreement with the investigator covers any fee that is to be paid to this principal, but it is not unusual that a separate contract is needed. The nature of these contracts vary according to local rules and legislation, but are generally intended to indemnify the principal against any increased costs brought about by the clinical trial.

The basis for the contract is usually some sort of collation of procedures above and beyond the normal routine, along with their costs. This can include extra physician and nurse visits, laboratory tests and even any hand-

The carrying through

ling costs billed by the pharmacy. Procedures which the patient must naturally undergo as a part of routine care is normally not compensated, but again, this can differ from country to country and institution to institution. Given the background information about extra resources and their costs, the principal and the sponsor reaches an agreement concerning compensation. The investigator has a key role, being the one who can best advice what is included in *normal* medical routine and what is not.

A patient's participation in a clinical trial must be entirely free of charge. Exceptions to this may occur sometimes in very large intervention studies in which the patients on the whole are treated according to current treatment practice. The patients may have to pay the regular patient fee for the consultation in such cases.

Insurance

The local legislation on insurance for patients or healthy subjects treated within clinical trials differ around the world. Though there are countries were there exists a nationwide insurance for any drug injuries, it is most common to rely on the insurance provided by the sponsor.

All pharmaceutical companies carry insurance that will indemnify patients for injuries occurred as an effect of participation in a clinical trial. Although there can be slight variations the general terms are very similar in most insurance policies, and the sponsor can provide ethical committees, authorities etc. with more information if requested.

Multi-center trials

Multi-center trials are studies that are run at more than one center. This can mean anything from two participating clinics to several hundred. These kinds of trials are becoming increasingly common, especially in an epidemiological context and for large intervention studies such as anti-hypertensive therapy's preventative effect in cardiovascular disease. Such studies can by definition not be done in one single center. Yet it is not only in these large contexts that multicenter studies appear. Regular studies are increasingly carried out at more than one center and for the phase III studies intended to document general safety and efficacy in a representative patient population, multi-center is the norm.

How the centers are chosen for a multicenter trial is a chapter in itself that entails an huge number of various motives. It may be that a disease is so rare that virtually all the clinics in a country having these patients are contacted. On other occasions there may be a special enthusiast who puts the whole thing into motion and simply chooses colleagues that he or she likes to work with. Sometimes a certain level of health care is desired, such as outpatient centers or home nursing care. The sponsor may wish to work with a well-know person in the field or simply select someone that they have had good working relationships with in the past. And some particularly large studies may even advertise for interested investigators.

In principle, multicenter trials are run in the exact same way as all other trials, but the fact that there are many participants involved can make some elements additionally complicated.

First and foremost a lot of discussion may arise concerning the writing of the protocol. Routines may vary among clinics, and each participant may have her own idea about how some elements should be performed. It is best to realize from the beginning that compromise will be needed. It is wisest that one or a few persons be delegated to write the protocol, and let all participants have a few rounds of submitting comments, and if possible have a meeting in which everyone agrees on the final draft. After that the protocol should not be revised unless it is made absolutely necessary for scientific or practical reasons, and those participants who do not accept the protocol should be allowed to withdraw from participating – the act of further revising infallibly leads to additional problems, more dissatisfied investigators etc. And this can get even more complicated if it is an international study, which is becoming increasingly common. In which case several countries' varying views need to be merged together, and is something that never happens without considerable effort.

The protocol should place special emphasis on how to ensure that all investigators act in accord. This can involve such simple matters as measuring blood pressure and checking liver enzymes. Should the variable in question be one of the main variables to be analyzed for the study, some time must be spent discussing the risk of between-clinic variation. Is everyone using the same type of blood compression cuff? Does everyone measure pressure the same way? Do all the labs use the same methods for AST and ALT? In some case the solution may be to let all the analyses of a certain type be carried out by a single lab. This gives good uniformity, and often functions optimally, but some new practical problems must then be resolved, such as how to ship the samples. The protocol should also state whether there is an intention to check if the variable measurements vary by center, and what is to be done about it if they do. Sometimes things may get so unlucky that an entire study cannot be successfully analyzed because one or two investigators deviate too much from the others in some way.

One good way to ensure that participants are working in accord during the study is to hold regular "investigators' meetings" with all investigators, or if the project is huge, all participants in the same region. These meetings should be made obligatory, especially for long-term studies. They provide the opportunity to exchange experiences with other investigators, discuss practical problems, and resolve any new problem while at an early stage. Additionally, it is often fun to meet colleagues, and anticipation does wonders for speeding up the enrollment in the time just preceding the meeting etc. When a sponsor exists, it is most suitably the sponsor's lot to organize these meetings. Of course it is possible to run a multicenter trial without these investigator meetings, but it increases the risk of variability and is not recommended.

Another aspect requiring a lot of consideration in multicenter trials is how the randomization of subjects is to be carried out. In double-blind drug studies, the randomization can be made in advance and the patients receive their numbered, anonymous medicine without any further procedure being needed. Studies testing different types of therapies can be a bit more complicated. Sometimes it is suitable to have a center that the investigator can call to receive the randomization. This method can ensure that the randomization is evenly distributed across all centers in the entire study, and in addition it provides a good overview of the study's progress. An international study might experience some difficulty with such a procedure due to time zones, which is another thing that has to be resolved before the study begins.

Data collection, monitoring, and quality control must, of course, be carried out identically in all clinical trials. The size of the multicenter study makes this a major undertaking, and it is not at all uncommon that several persons are needed to do follow-ups in very large projects, which may be taking place in several countries at the same time. Anyone running a large multicenter trial as the principal investigator without a sponsor should be fully aware that this is a heavy responsibility and a lot of work. The ICH GCP guidelines open the possibility of running certain types of studies without direct monitoring, but this must be well motivated in the protocol, and approved by the ethics committees and regulatory authorities, if applicable.

Once the trials is completed and analyzed comes the next problem: writing the report. Who should be the author? Who else should be included as co-authors? Whose name will come first?

Once again the recommendation is that this should be determined in advance and stated in the protocol. Sometimes an initiating enthusiast is chosen as the first name, but more often there are several researchers who have completed the work together, and thus there must be agreement over who does what, the ranking of names etc. Many times this group may be listed as the author. In large studies there is no way that all participants can be listed as authors and it is important that all are in agreement over this. However, every participant's name should be stated somewhere in the article, such as in a "list of participating investigators" (see also "Publication").

Despite all these practical problems, multicenter trials are becoming more common for the simple reason that they often give results much faster than single center studies, and that is something all involved benefit from.

Study documentation

The following documents are required prior to starting a clinical trial.

- The study protocol signed by the investigator and sponsor.
- A Curriculum Vitae for each participating investigator and also for other persons having defined duties in the study (in the case of medical devices, the CV must be attested).
- Curriculum Vitae for the head of laboratories included in the study (only some studies – see "IND studies") or laboratories certificate number, or similar.
- A list of normal values for each participating laboratory and documentation of testing procedures.
- A list of names of the staff who will be involved in the study along with their stated function, and if necessary combined with:
- A signature/delegation list with signatures of those persons holding the right to enter the required data in the CRF.
- An application to and permission from the relevant ethics committee.
- An application to and permission from the regulatory authority, if applicable.
- Patient information and consent forms (and if appropriate, all recruiting advertisements).
- Any staff information.

- The Case Report Form.
- Drug Accountability Form plus examples of labeling.
- Instructions for handling the drugs or medical devices.
- The individual code envelope (if appropriate).
- The contract between the sponsor and responsible principal (if appropriate) and/or the investigator or institution.
- Investigator's brochure or its equivalent.
- Monitoring report(s) from the preliminary visit at the center.

Any clinical trial intended for submission to the FDA may require additional documentation (see "IND studies").

During and after the study

Finding suitable patients

Suitable patients are usually considerably more difficult to find than is first believed. Not only must they pass all inclusion and exclusion criteria, and consent to the study, but they must also be deemed likely to complete the study. At this point there is a dilemma. In order to get as representative patients as possible, subjective selection methods must be used extremely sparingly. The ideal is to consecutively enroll all patients who pass the criteria. In reality it is impossible to deny that subjective evaluations about the patients' suitability plays a role. One way of later seeing whether the sample is representative or not is to keep a log during the enrollment period that covers every patient not included in the study, but still having the disease being investigated. Simple demographic data plus the reason why the patient was excluded can provide good material for future evaluation. In some countries local rules even require that the protocol describes which procedures will be used for registering and subsequently evaluating those patients who were excluded from the study.

The overriding point here is that finding suitable patients can often be much tougher than anticipated. Making up a list of possible patients already from the initial planning stages can greatly facilitate matters. It may also provide a much more realistic idea about the true pool of candidates. In this connection, a computerized patient database searchable by diagnosis can be a very valuable asset.

One of the best ways to form an opinion about the realistic incoming supply of patients is to perform a real live test. During the time that the protocol is being discussed and while waiting for start-up authorizations, apply the inclusion and exclusion criteria to the patients that do come in and write down how may these are, whether they could have been asked to participate or why not etc. This provides a good estimate of what proportion of all candidates might be approachable for inclusion. In chronic diseases this also provides a pool of suitable patients that can subsequently be contacted for possible enrollment.

Delegating tasks and responsibility

It is the investigator's responsibility that the study adheres to the protocol, that the patients be medically treated in the correct manner, and that the information entered into the CRF is accurate.

However, there are many situations where it is possible to delegate responsibility for certain parts of the study to other persons. Specially employed research assistants or research nurses can be very acceptable in this context. But, it must be made very clear which duties are being delegated, and a system for regular monitoring of these duties should be implemented in order to avoid confusion. This transfer of responsibility must be put in writing; for example, on a signature and delegation list and can also be written into the protocol or an appendix.

Exactly which responsibilities may be delegated must be determined from study to study and country to country; however, decisions that affect the patient's continued treatment and safety (continued participation in the trial, alteration in dosage, etc.) must be made by the investigator.

Monitoring

Monitoring is that which the sponsor (or principal investigator when there is no sponsor) does during the course of the study to ensure for himself and the study participants that everything is going correctly and according to plan. Companies are required to have written rules about the how the monitoring is supposed to be done (see "SOP" and "The Clinical Trial Monitor"). A monitoring visit consists of a representative from the sponsor, usually the clinical monitor, paying a visit to the clinic, partly in to order to review the study's progress and partly to create an opportunity to exchange information. The frequency of these visits depends on the nature of the study and the timetable, but should not occur too infrequently. A relatively common visiting rate is every 4th to 8th week. It is necessary for the investigator to be present at these visits in order to answer questions, check the data in the patient charts etc. Other staff members may at times be required to attend, particularly when a research nurse or other person has been specially assigned to run parts of the study. Sometimes the clinical monitor wants to talk to other staff members too, but this request is usually submitted in advance.

It may occasionally seem burdensome to set aside time for these visits; nonetheless, frequent visits should be encouraged. These visits present the opportunity for an "outside" person to review the recorded information and thereby considerably increases the chance that mistakes and misunderstandings may be discovered. This saves time and effort in the long run.

The following points are generally reviewed during a visit:

The study's progress
- How many patients have been enrolled, withdrawn or completed?
- Have the patients been informed and given their consent?
- Is the timetable being held? If not, what can be done?

The protocol
- Has it been followed or has a mistake sneaked in or misunderstanding occurred?

The Case Report Form
- Have they been filled in? Is anything missing?
- Is the information in agreement with the original data (determined by sampling)?

Adverse events and reactions
- Has anything unforeseen appeared?
- Have they all been recorded correctly?

The study drug or device
- Is the supply sufficient?
- Is the drug or device being correctly handled? If not, what can be done?

Staff and related resources
- Has any new person appeared who might require additional information?
- Has the size of the staff and other resources remained the same? If not, what can be done?

General
- Have any problems occurred?

It is especially important at the start of the study to have frequent monitoring visits. It is on these early occasions that systematic errors and unforeseen practical obstacles in the protocol are discovered, and also when there is the greatest risk that the protocol is not being correctly followed. The monitor is required to write a report about all visits; the fact that a visit has occurred must also be documented; for example, by the clinic maintaining a visitors list that is countersigned by the investigator or other coworker. Any decision that has been made, or an action that has been done – or needs to be done – should be documented in writing and sent to the investigator.

In addition to the monitoring visits, other representatives from the sponsor may pay a visit. This may be a case of verifying whether the sponsor's internal verification system for guaranteeing high-quality trials (known as "quality assurance") is functioning (see "Audits, inspections and quality assurance").

Adverse events – Side-effects and other events

"Adverse events" is a concept used for classifying not only drug-related adverse reactions but also other events that happen during the course of a trial. This applies to such widely separated events as a common cold or a death due to accident. This concept differs from what doctors commonly refer to as "side-effects" and it needs to be emphasized that it also includes things that don't necessarily seem to be related with the treatment. Everything that happens to a patient during a study must be documented, regardless of whether it might be connected to the treatment or not. When the results from a large study are finally assembled it may turn out that that which appeared as a random event turns out to follow some sort of pattern. Pharmaceutical companies are required to have an established routine about how various types of incidents and adverse effects are to be recorded and sent to the companies, and this routine is usually described in the protocol. For "banal" incidents or adverse effects it is usually sufficient to merely document these in the patient charts. However, serious adverse events or reactions must be separately recorded and immediately reported to the sponsor within 24 hours. A telephone call is sufficient for the first contact but must be followed by a written report. There are regulations for applicable time limitations and these must be stated in the protocol.

Serious adverse events are any untoward occurrences that:

• result in death,
• arc life-threatening,
• requires inpatient hospitalization or prolongation of existing hospitalization
• results in persistent or significant disability/incapacity
or
• are a congenital anomalies/birth defect

Accordingly, it is important that the sponsor immediately be informed about such events in order to discern as quickly as possible any potentially negative trend. Timetables are usually set up so that these events must be reported to the sponsor within 24 hours from the time that the investigator is made aware of them.

An adverse reaction that is both serious and unexpected (and thus can also be suspected of being possibly caused by the study drug used) must in most countries also be submitted by the investigator to the regulatory authority and/or ethical committee (according to local regulations) within 15 working days from the date that it occurred. The sponsor is to report the same patient to the same bodies within 15 working days from the time that the investigator was made aware of the case. At this time the sponsor identifies the patient using the patient identification number and the study designation, and in this way double registration can be avoided. If the unexpected, serious adverse reaction is fatal or life threatening, it must be reported within seven days by both the investigator and the sponsor.

Both the investigator and the sponsor are also required to report in a similar timely manner if they detect a suspicious increase in frequency or degree of severity of known adverse reactions or incidents, and that could possibly affect the design or performance of the study.

In addition to the reports directly submitted when the events occurred, the sponsor is also obliged to submit an annual account for serious adverse reactions or incidents that lead to the study drug being prematurely withdrawn. At the end of the study in the final report, a summation of all observed adverse reactions and incidents must be given; this is in addition to the serious adverse reactions and incidents already reported.

There is an additional reporting obligation on the sponsor to report all serious adverse reactions that occurred in other nations to the pertinent authorities in countries were studies are ongoing within a specified time period. This is also true when there is a suspected increase in the number and severity of already know adverse effects. The sponsor must also regularly update the investigator about these adverse events.

Audits, inspections and quality assurance

In principle, any clinical trial at all may be subjected to a later audit or inspection. An audit or inspection are virtually the same thing, but it is called an audit when it is performed by the company and an inspection when carried out by a governmental authority. The USA has a long-established program in which the regulatory authorities use both sampling and "for cause" inspections. These most often target key studies required for drug registration ("pivotal studies") or studies being performed by investigators who have previously be known to have not completely lived up to the requirements of Good Clinical Practice. The FDA also conduct inspections in other counties should the crucial studies be performed abroad. Other national regulatory authorities also carry out inspections, but generally only within their own country, at least so far.

Whether an audit or inspection, these checks look at virtually everything affecting the study. At the sponsor, one examines whether the study was documented, followed up and reported correctly. At the clinic the focus is on the verification of the archiving, documentation, patient consent, reporting of drug accountability, and of course, original data. Special emphasis is usually directed on whether the patient's consent was handled correctly, that all original data was saved and kept available, and that they agree with what is recorded in the patient's CRF. The regulatory authority of the own country is a supervising authority and thus normally has legal access to the patient charts automatically; however, if a foreign authority requests to directly review these charts, the patient's consent is required in many countries (see "Ensuring the patient's confidentiality"). Should an audit or inspection happen in a study, it is best to set aside considerable working time to resolve this – up to a week of full time work for large studies.

The audits that a company conducts on its own studies are a part of the system for assessing the quality it desires and is often called "quality assurance" or something similar. These systems are intended as guarantees that studies are performed correctly, including, for example, checks that the investigator did the work properly. This audit is generally carried out by a person employed by the sponsor but who has not been involved in the project and belongs to an independent organization within the company. In this case, control of the original data and procedures are usually as strict as those carried out by an authority. An audit is not normally conducted for each investigator, but the more important the study, or the greater the number of patients enrolled, the greater is the "risk" – or perhaps "opportunity" – of being audited.

There is now considerable experience about what these controls have shown around the world, both for audits and inspections. In general it may be said that the standard is fairly high, but some problems keep coming up repeatedly. The most common are the difficulty in identifying which version of the protocol is actually in force, uncertainty about how and when the patient's informed consent was obtained in relation to when the patients actually entered the study, insufficient accounting for the drugs used, incomplete data entries into the Case Report Forms and archiving of the original data. Nor is it completely uncommon that one of the participating centers in a multi-center study has forgotten to submit its application to the Ethics Committee or regulatory authority; and there are often failures in submitting major amendments to the protocol to the same bodies. Finally and unfortunately, there is a common carelessness about sending yearly or final reports to the Ethics Committee and/or authorities.

Carelessness and fraud in clinical trials

Unfortunately, in this context, some more dismal aspects concerning clinical trials needs to be discussed, namely carelessness and willful misrepresentation – i.e. fraud. It is, of course, not so that clinical research has been spared from this phenomenon. It has also become more public in recent years, especially some spectacular US and English cases of fraud by established and well-known researchers within both pharmaceutical and purely scientific research.

The most common reason for erroneous data is nonetheless carelessness, even if it sometimes can be difficult to draw the line between carelessness and pure cheating. However, proper monitoring during the course of the study should be able to discover this early on and see to corrections.

It is much harder to deal with deliberate fraud. There are a number of known cases around the world, and experts in the area make an estimate that perhaps as much as 1% of investigators cheat in some way, both within and outside of pharmaceutical research; meaning that the problem cannot be wished away.

When should fraud be suspected? One of the basic prerequisites is that studies be correctly monitored using thoroughly trained persons. Discovery is often a case of one's experience and common sense leading one to begin smelling a rat. Perhaps it is a case of the data looking too good: all the patients come to every treatment visit, take all of their tablets and no one experiences an adverse event etc. Perhaps all the returned drug packages look untouched, or perhaps all the data in the CRFs are written with the same pen, despite the fact that visits occur every third month.

Thoroughly thought-out and well-executed fraud is not easily discovered, so what is to be done when there is suspicion of a "smelly rat"? If there is a corporate sponsor, probably the first thing to occur will be an audit. Perhaps the company will request – officially or otherwise – that the regulatory agency inspect the investigator involved. When there is no sponsor, or if it is case of non-drug related research, everything become a bit less clear. In some countries (like UK, Denmark and Sweden) there now exists independent investigational bodies to turn to, should one suspect fraud. These bodies can conduct an investigation to ascertain whether a fraud has indeed occurred, and can also recommend, and in the UK, execute suitable repercussions. There have for instance been cases were the physicians license to practice medicine has been withdrawn. However, in many countries such bodies do not exist, and other ways need to be found.

Every pharmaceutical company should have a specific SOP concerning how suspected fraud should be handled, investigated, and reported to the regulatory authority, ethics committee and anyone else involved.

If fraud has been convincingly demonstrated in a clinical drug trial, the ethics committee and the relevant authority must be informed. The occurrence of fraud may have great consequence for the study, which may be declared invalid in its entirety. In the US, fraud is subject to legal prosecution, and the information that the investigator has committed such offense or has received warnings is made public.

Documentation and archiving

Both the investigator and the sponsor must document and archive everything concerning the study. This is motivated by reasons of safety and reasons of verification, having the necessary information at hand in case of an examination of the study at some future date. The documentation must be kept in a secure manner such that unauthorized person are denied access to it.

The necessary items to be archived are those things required for being able to reconstruct the trial at a future date and usually consist of:

- a copy of the study protocol with any amendments and revisions
- a copy of the most recent Investigators Brochure and list of which Investigators Brochure was applicable during each phase of the study
- an updated Curriculum Vitae of each participant
- copies of applications to and authorization from regulatory authorities, ethics committees and sponsors
- copies of information for patients and documentation of informed consent
- signature and delegation lists
- copies of the CRFs
- copy of documents concerning drug accountability
- documentation concerning adverse events encountered
- all original data from the study
- annual and final reports about the study
- a list of the patients' identity with respect to the patient identification number used.

In addition sponsors archive everything that shows how the study was conducted and supervised – such as monitoring and auditing reports.

These document must be retained until at least two years after the drug or device has received its final approval in an ICH region and such that no further authorizations will be sought. Naturally, no investigator can be expected to keep track of this, which means that the sponsor is responsible for informing an investigator when archiving is no longer necessary. If the documents are to be moved, or if the investigator moves elsewhere, the sponsor must be informed in writing and told where the documents are now located and who has assumed responsibility for their storage. It is especially important to keep the patient's identity list in a secure place.

The term "original data" covers all data collected for a patient during the study. Patient charts with patient history data, lab results, EKGs, radiology findings, nurse comments etc., etc. Especially important are data concerning the study's efficacy variables. It is important to keep in mind that it is the raw data itself, such as the actual ECG strip and not its interpretation that should be added to the patient's medical chart.

Archiving this original data is extremely important. This data is the basis for the study results, and the archiving aims at enabling verification of the results afterwards. Remember that the sponsor does not have a copy of this original data, and thus it is crucial that the data be stored in a secure manner. It is fully possible to keep this data in the patient's medical chart provided that there are fail-safe methods for storing this information in its entirety.

The investigator's copy of the CRFs must also be stored for the same time period. This is preferably done by the investigator, but the investigator can contract (in writing!) with the sponsor about archiving the forms on behalf of the investigator.

4 Processing results

Data and computer processing

Today virtually every study's results are analyzed by computer in one way or another. According to international laws on computer usage, limits have been established about how databases using personal information may be set-up and what they may contain. Even though these rules vary somewhat between different countries the general basics are quite similar. Databases containing information about a person's identity and civic national registry numbers are not to be made available to any other person than specified medical care employees, and such registers may not be established without authorization. The sponsor will often assist with the data processing, and the computer registers created for this purpose must be completely anonymous. The sponsor must also receive authorization in order to establish these computer databases. In many countries including the member states of the EU, the sponsor is also required to obtain permission for transferring said data to another country, this includes the transmission of handwritten data in CRFs, instead of electronically, and for which complete anonymity is a strict requirement. The same demands are incumbent on an individual investigator, of course, who may require that the data be physically transferred from one site to another.

The person establishing a database has additional things to consider. There must be secure protection against outsiders gaining access to the system. The system being used should of course be dependable, validated and have documented user instructions. Control and adequate back-up systems are required, and finally those granted access to the data must be competent and specified (that is, stated on an authorized user's list).

Analysis of results

Before analyzing the study's result, it is necessary to ensure as best one can that the database is complete and accurate. The CRFs are reviewed and an attempt is made to complete any missing data or correct erroneous ones before any analysis is begun, and especially before any codes are broken. There is sometimes a matter of interpretation about how some of the efficacy or safety test results are to be evaluated. Hopefully, this has been foreseen and the proper procedures have been clearly stated in the protocol. If this is not the case, it becomes important to confer with all participating investigators and reach agreement about how these interpretations are to be resolved, and carry this out before anyone is made aware of the patient's membership in a study treatment group. The standard case in double-blind studies is that the codes are not broken before all the results are evaluated and statistically analyzed. The time point when the codes are broken, and by whom, must be recorded. The codes may be broken in two stages, in which the study group membership is first revealed as "A" or "B," for example. All statistical analyses and comparison are completed, and afterwards the final code is then broken. This procedure is often called "triple-blind".

It is more difficult to objectively supplement and control the database in open studies. There is a clear risk for bias. Asking for the assistance of colleagues who are not otherwise involved in the study may help considerably.

It is very often the sponsor who carries out the statistical work, because they generally have much greater expertise and resources in this respect. This is, of course, quite proper and usually of great assistance. But it should be kept in mind that the investigator thereby loses a certain amount of control of the information. Not that the data will be misrepresented or altered, but rather it is always more difficult to influence the type of analysis, manner of presentation etc., if the investigator has no direct contact with the statistician doing the analysis. The best solution is for the investigator and the sponsor to discuss together what is to be analyzed, and how, at an early enough stage to be specified in the protocol. Once the agreed-upon analyses have been completed, a discussion can be begun about possible additional analyses.

Publication

The most important advice on publication is that this should be fully determined in advance! The protocol should state which reserved rights both the sponsor and/or investigator have when approaching publication. This usually means that each has a mutual obligation to allow the other party to review upcoming publications – before they are submitted – and to allow a reasonable time period for this. It may also be wise to make a contract about ownership rights of the resultant data; that is, can the investigator and/or sponsor refuse publication? Otherwise the answer to that question is "no," neither the investigator and/or sponsor can refuse. However, there may be completely legitimate views concerning when and how, and this should be discussed in advance. Concerning multicenter trials, it may also be necessary to describe the order in which the total results and any sub-studies may be published.

The authorship of the main article and report, and whose name is to appear first should there be more than one investigator, should also be discussed in advance. In some cases the investigator has both the time and skill to do both the analyses and write the report afterwards. More often, the sponsor does the analyses and even compiles a report of the results.

There are two main types of reports. The first is a full report sent to the regulatory authority for the purpose of drug registration, the other is the usual scientific paper.

A registration report is a comprehensive document with a detailed review of the material, methods and results and having extensive appendices containing data in tabulated form. These reports are written following specific templates, and it is the sponsor who usually puts these together.

The scientific papers are considerably more concise, yet still must contain sufficient information for allowing the reader to form an opinion about the reliability of the results. The composition of reliable and readable papers is a noble art that can scarcely be learned on the fly. The majority of journals have writers' guidelines that show how that particular journal wants the paper formatted. In short, the paper has to explain why the study was performed, how it was done, what the results were, and how the author(s) interpreted them. The principle is that so much information is given about the procedures used that someone else could replicate the study and (hopefully) come to the same results.

This handbook does not intend to give exhaustive writing instructions, but a few details can be named. As emphasized above, informed consent must be granted by each patient, and that this occurred ought to be stated. The ethics committee actually authorizing the study should be named. The majority of journals will not publish papers on studies that were not carried out in compliance with the Helsinki Declaration. There should also be a description of which statistical tests were employed. The patients who couldn't complete the study are as important as those who did – at the very least – and should be carefully reviewed. The paper should also report whether the study was sponsored by a company or some other party.

Many papers are submitted in English, and if possible, it is a good idea that even those feeling secure in this skill allow an English language expert to review the paper. Poor wording can lead to a humorous impression and unnecessarily attract attention away from the actual results. A final word of advice; confirm that the conclusion stated in the body of the text is in agreement with that stated as the goal in the beginning of the paper.

Unfortunately, it is often hard to get "negative" findings published; that is, studies finding no appreciable advantages for the (new) treatment method under study. This is unfortunate because it renders the possibility of reaching a balanced view of this treatment method more difficult. Even if the study results in "negative findings" an accurate report must be written for sending to the authorities and for other uses.

5 Conclusion

Overview and time perspectives

The many activities involved in planning and performing a clinical trial are often carried out simultaneously. Some activities require that others tasks have been completed first, and it isn't always easy to keep control over all the various factors. The following flowchart is an attempt to highlight the important stages in a common clinical trial, beginning with the original idea and continuing on to the report and archiving. As can be seen it is the period between the time that a decision has been made to do the study and the time that the study actually begins that requires the greatest number of simultaneous activities, and a vast number of details that must be organized. Once the study actually gets underway the activities generally follow each other in sequence, except for the monitoring and quality control that are carried out throughout the entire course of the study (see Fig. 1).

How much time does it all take? Unfortunately the answer is almost always "more time than you think". The following diagram [Fig. 2] is an overview of the how the same steps that were presented in Fig. 1 can spread out over time. This hypothetical trial can be considered a relatively simple trial covering 4 to 6 weeks of treatment on 20 patients having a relatively common complaint.

It is best to count on 6 months of time from the time that the idea is hatched until the study actually starts – provided that nothing happens to delay the timetable. It is possible for this to take less time, but it can take considerably more time if the protocol is complicated and needs to be discussed with several participating investigators, to name just two examples. During this time there are many other practical details to be worked out in addition to filing applications to the ethics committee and regulatory authority.

Once the study is to start, patients must be enrolled. All the potential patients that were around just a week before have a curious habit of totally

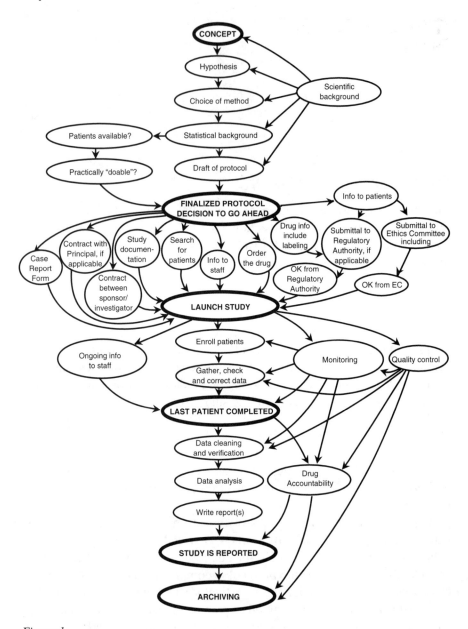

Figure 1

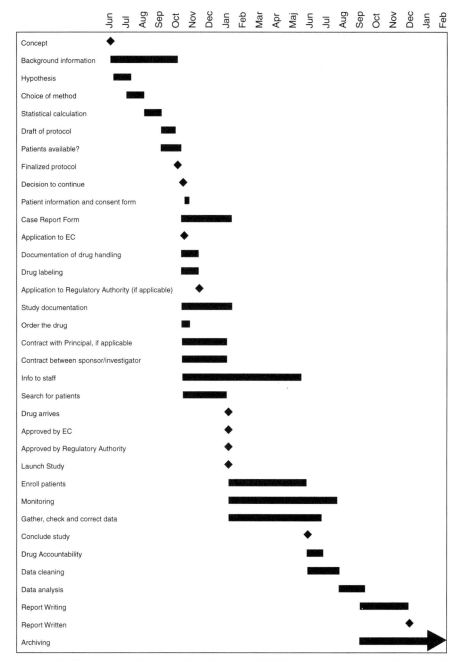

Figure 2 Whole page time schedule listing all (35) steps on the vertical axis and timetable on the horizontal, sorted by sequence of execution.

vanish when the time finally comes. Sitting there studying the inclusion and exclusion criteria reveals why so many potential subjects drop out of consideration – and after that, those who remain also have to consent to the whole thing. If one has used the planning time to go through potential patients and have them lined up in ones mind the enrollment can be considerably quicker, of course.

Once the study is over and the last patient has completed therapy, verification and supplementation of data takes place – a very time consuming process. Hopefully one has done most of this continuously during the progress of the study so that there should only remain a small amount of issues to clarify after the last patient has completed, but that is unfortunately not always the case. Next comes data processing, analyses and last but not least the writing of the report and/or article. Following that comes archiving, and not until then is the trial truly over. In our hypothetical trial the whole process takes one and a half years – and this is definitely not a worst case scenario (see Fig. 2).

Conclusion

Many of medicine's greatest achievements in recent years have depended on the development of new, more effective drugs, medical devices and other aids to clinical treatment. Countless lives have been saved and suffering alleviated. The only way to develop new drugs and related products and finding their proper place in the therapy arsenal is through well-conducted clinical trials. It ought to be natural, perhaps even mandatory, for all doctors to participate in clinical trials, but unfortunately this isn't the case. Completing a clinical trial requires interest, time, resources and patience. If these preconditions exist, and if the opportunity arises, then participating in a clinical trial is heartily recommended. The act of participating provides an invaluable insight into how this type of research is conducted. In addition to improved and new skills, one also receives understanding about research's possibilities and pitfalls. This, in its turn, enables a much improved skill in the ability to evaluate the validity other research findings that can affect the physician's own choice of therapies.

Hopefully, all this will lead to that which every doctor desires, and as the Helsinki Declaration underlines is obliged to strive for, namely, providing every patient with the best possible care.

References and literature cited

Laws, ordinance and directions:
Health and Human Services Dept., FDA. 1) Protection of human subjects, informed consent, Institutional Review Boards; Federal Register, vol. 46, No 17, 27/1/81.
FDA's Bioresearch Monitoring Programme, F. O. Kelsey; Methods and Findings in Experimental Clinical Pharmacology. 4, 503–8 (1982).

Guidelines, etc.:
Guidelines for Good Clinical Practice. ICH Harmonised Tripartite Guideline.
Good Clinical Practice for Trials on Medicinal Products in the European Community. (111/3976/88-EN)

Literature:
Clinical trials – a practical approach. S. J. Pocock (1983). John Wiley and Sons Ltd., ISBN 0-471-90155-5.
Guide to clinical trials. B. Spilker (1991). Raven Press.
Uniform requirements for Manuscripts submitted to Biomedical Journals; Brit. Med. Journal and Annals of Internal Medicine, June 1982.
Organise a multicenter trial, C. Warlow, Br. Med. J. 300:180–183 (1990).

Appendix I – Suggestions for drawing up a protocol

1. Study Synopsis

Presents a short summary of the primary concepts in the study, preferably no more than a full page. State the object of the investigation, who the patients will be as well as how many, the duration and type of treatment to be administered, and how the study is to be evaluated.

2. Background and rationale

Describes the background and rationale for the entire study. Reference may be made to earlier published data and the treatments they describe, especially the newest ones. If relevant, postulate the theory to be tested and why the new treatment form is to be tested.

3. Objective

Describes the study's primary goals and any secondary goals. This section should be kept to one or very few sentences – the objective of the study should be clearly and concisely expressed. Complicated and, especially, numerous research objectives often lead to no results at all.

4. Subjects and methods

4.1 Study design

Describes the design of the study: e.g., whether it is to be a double-blind, randomized multi-center study, or some other form.

4.2 Selection of subjects

This section may suitably be divided into four parts: The inclusion criteria, the exclusion criteria, a statement on the number of patients to be included (the rationale for the number chosen is usually presented in the statistics section further along in the protocol) and if and how notations are to be recorded for those patients not included in the trial.

The inclusion criteria are usually few in number; for example, that the patients in the study in question should be between 18 and 65 years old, have the intended disease as defined by some standard criteria and volunteer their participation.

The exclusion criteria often become rather numerous, something that may considerably hinder the performance of the study. These criteria should be minimized to the absolute number needed, and primarily those affecting safety aspects are to be retained; for example pregnancy, lactation, contraindications to certain treatment forms, allergy to the medicine being used etc. It is also common to exclude [drug and alcohol] abusers. In order to gain an understanding about whether the patients included in the study are representative or not, information about those patients who are not included should be recorded in some manner. This may take the form of a logbook covering all potential candidates, reporting their initials, age, sex, and specific reasons for why any particular patient was excluded from the study.

4.3 Study drugs, treatment methods and other aids included in the trial

A great deal of information is to be included in this section. Name the drugs to be used, their dosage, mode of administration and treatment intervals. The choice of dose must be explained. State how the drugs are to be made "blind," that is how they are to made identical in appearance, or whether any other solution to this problem is to be used. Include the same type of information, dosage etc., for placebo if used. At times, the study drug used must be titrated according to the patient's response to the treatment, and thus careful rules for how this is to be done must be included. There should also be a statement about how the dose is to be reduced in the case of adverse effects or excessively pronounced effect.

One section should be devoted to the practical aspects of administering the drug. Packaging size, how frequently used, its labeling and use is to be reviewed.

Concerning medical devices, there must be usage instructions in the native language covering usage, maintenance and cleaning. The protocol must also describe the contents of these instructions and how they are to be furnished to the staff and patients.

Also state how the post-study treatment is to be conducted, especially in those cases where continuation of the study treatment seems desirable.

There should also be a statement on how the patient code may be broken, and what is to be done in the case of an acute situation.

4.4 Concomitant drugs

This section discusses what should be done with other medications that the patient may need during the study. Some medications may be contraindicated due to interactions with others, while others may be contraindicated if they influence the efficacy variable to be measured. In addition, some studies may require "rescue medication" on hand in case the study drug is insufficient; and these must be carefully described as well as their usage.

4.5 Treatment plan

Describe how the study is to be conducted in purely practical terms, visit be visit – what is to be done at each visit, the interval between visits, etc. For example, can the patients be considered in need of further treatment? Should any special samples be drawn? There must also be a discussion on what is to be done with patients who withdraw their participation for some reason.

4.6 Efficacy evaluation

All information on how the efficacy of the drug or devices should be gathered under this heading. This may include things like blood pressure measurements, specific lab tests, exercise stress test, ad nauseam. It is important to describe exactly how the tests are to be performed, even such routine tests as blood pressure measurement, and how the actual efficacy measure obtained is to be evaluated. A pre-established target of what constitutes a satisfactory result and what doesn't needs to be defined. Also state where the analysis of the efficacy variable is to be made. Are all tests to be performed at a single, central site? If these tests are to be conducted at each study site, describe how standardization is to be ensured.

4.7 Safety evaluation

This section describes the actions needed for evaluating the safety aspects. For example, should a special blood sample be drawn, or blood pressure measured, at certain occasions? Should these be taken before, after, or even before and after the study? Report here how adverse events are to be defined and recorded; and what actions are to be taken when adverse events of varying nature appear, especially serious adverse events and reactions.

This section may also be used for describing serious but expected incidents – for example, death due to cancer in oncology studies – that are not going to be reported separately during the study, but will be reported instead after the completion of the study in the evaluation of the results.

5. Statistics and data analysis

The statistics section may be divided into two parts, the planning stage and the descriptions of the outcome.

The planning contains the calculations that form the basis for the number of patients chosen given known facts or assumptions about the drug's efficacy.

The outcome section is a description of those variables to be evaluated, and which statistics will be used chosen. If an interim analysis must be performed, the method should be described in detail.

The section on data analysis generally discusses how the information is to be collected (ex., Case Report Forms), and how they are to be analyzed etc. Safety and quality aspects concerning the data management should also be included. This section is also a suitable one for describing which documentation will be needed during the study and how long it is to be kept.

6. Ethical and regulatory requirements

Since it is obligatory everywhere to apply to a research ethics for study approval, there is a tendency not to state this in the protocol. However, there should usually be a statement stating that it is the intention to follow the Helsinki Declaration and that the study will seek approval as described above. There should also be paragraph about the ethical considerations surrounding the current study.

You should state whether any additional insurance has been purchased for the study, above and beyond basic public health insurance, and whether the compensation is to be paid to the participants (besides travel costs, it is usually only healthy volunteer subjects who receive payment for participation).

Included here, or as an appendix, a copy of the written patient information and consent form should be included, along with descriptions on how consent is to be obtained and recorded. State as well that a patient identification list is to exist and how it is be archived.

7. Research administration

This section discusses such issues as how monitoring and quality controls are to be undertaken, how the Case Report Forms are to be handled, what the study's timetable looks like, whether investigator meetings are to occur etc.

Here, or at some other place in the protocol, a description should be written about how the staff is to be informed, and how any delegation or sharing of authority is going to be distributed among colleagues.

There should also be information on how the study documentation is to be archived.

8. Reports and publications

This section is to state who is to analyze the data and who is to compile and write reports and publications. The sponsor generally reserves the right of advanced review of articles for publication, along with a reasonable period to reply with comments (typically 30 days). The converse is also true, that the researcher has a right to comment on materials that the sponsors wants to publish (but not, however, the researcher's permission to use an already published article as a reference).

9. Signed agreement

Finally, there must be a page where the investigator and the sponsor both undersign that they are in agreement about how the study is to be conducted in relation to the protocol in question. In addition, and normally not included in the protocol, there should be a separate written contract between the investigator and the sponsor concerning financial and other matters.

10. Addenda

It is very common that addenda accompanies the protocol, such as a description of methods, detailed instructions on the reporting of adverse effects, copies of the information delivered to both staff and patients, the Helsinki Declaration, etc.

A necessary, and very practical, appendix is a flowchart of the study showing each visit and what is to be done during these; it should be written in tabular, or other easily comprehended, form. Depending on the native language at the site of the study, even if the protocol is in English, the flow-chart ought to be in the native language in order to assist staff members.

11. Reference list

Finally, include an appendix naming and identifying the references cited in the protocol.

Appendix II
– Glossary of common terms used in clinical research

ADE   Adverse Drug Event, any event that is unexpected and harmful or undesirable and occurring during the conduct of the clinical trial.

ADR   Adverse Drug Reaction, each reaction to a substance (or where such suspicion cannot be ruled out) that is unexpected and harmful or undesirable.

amendment   an addition or revision to the study protocol.

audit   a verification carried out by a pharmaceutical company and which is a systematic and independent examination to determine whether a clinical study is being correctly conducted and reported.

base-line   the time point at the start of the study, often the occasion against which the study's results are compared.

bias   a predetermined perception or a condition that affects the results or the interpretation of a study, such that it no longer is in agreement with the truth.

CDP   Clinical Development Plan, an overriding plan for the development of a new medical substance or product.

CDS   Core Data Sheet. A description of a drugkey properties, effects, adverse reaction profile etc. An equivalent to the European Summary of Product Characteristic (SmPC).

CRA   Clinical Research Associate, commonly used for the clinical monitor or assistant monitor.

CRF   Case Report Form (or Case Record Form), the form on which all data needed for evaluation of the study is recorded and collected.

CRM	Clinical Research Manager, usually another name for the clinical monitor or senior clinical monitor.
CRO	Contract Research Organization, an independent company or organization that conducts clinical trials on behalf of the sponsor.
CTX	Clinical Trial Exemption, an application for a clinical trial in the UK.
CV	Curriculum vitae, a résumé of the training and experience of a given person.
carry-over effect	lingering effect from a previous treatment.
center	the place (clinic, ward etc.) where the clinical trial is conducted.
clean file	When all information from a study is controlled, corrected and supplemented. When a clean file is obtained, the statistical analysis may begin.
co-investigator	investigator; a physician or dentist who participates in a clinical trial and bears responsibility that the trial is performed correctly, but does not carry the formal head responsibility at the clinic in question. (cf. "sub-investigator").
compliance	cooperation, the patients' actual performance in adhering to the instruction on how to take the drug; or the physician's adherence to the protocol and GCP regulations.
control	verification, also a term used for those patients who receive a reference drug, no treatment, placebo treatment or the like.
cross-over	a study design where each patient, in random order, is treated with all the preparations being used in a study.
drop out	a patient who doesn't complete the study in accordance with the protocol.

double blind	neither the patient nor investigating team knows which treatment the patient is receiving at the time of treatment.
double dummy	a techniques used for blinding when two comparative drugs can not be made to look identical. An identical placebo of each drug is then manufactured and all patients receive tablets of both drugs – an active tablet of drug A, an inactive of drug B or vice versa.
drug accountability	an accounting of all the drugs that were used in the trial, from the company to the patient then back to the clinic and finally to the company again, and to destruction of any remaining drug.
editing	review of the CRF or other basal data as a preparation for entering the data into a computer.
end-point	an event or marker that is measured for studying efficacy or safety. For example, an observed myocardial infarction or a given value on a biochemical lab test.
expiry date	the date of expiration of the drug.
FDA	the Food and Drug Administration, the US drug regulatory authority.
GCP	Good Clinical Practice, the authorities' requirements and guidelines for how clinical trials are to be conducted.
GLP	Good Laboratory Practice, the authorities' requirements and guidelines for how laboratory work is to be conducted.
GMP	Good Manufacturing Practice, the authorities' requirements and guidelines for how drugs are to be produced.
IND	Investigational New Drug, a US term for new medicinal compounds being tested and their development programs.

IND application	an application in the US for initiating a defined research program containing clinical trials for evaluation of a new drug.
informed consent	consent of the patient to participate in the study after having received comprehensive written and verbal information about the study, any associated risks, advantages, and that participation is entirely voluntary.
inspection	a verification carried out by regulatory authorities of data, procedures and documentation of the studies carried out. Usually takes place at the investigator site, but may be conducted at the sponsor, CRO or its equivalent. (See "audit" for the company's corresponding action.)
intention-to-treat or "intent to treat"	an analysis where all randomized patients are or included in the final analysis regardless of whether they completed the study correctly or not.
interim analysis	a planned or unplanned analysis of the results while the study is still ongoing.
investigator	a physician or dentist involved in conducting a clinical trial.
Investigators Brochure	a summary of the knowledge surrounding a drug produced by the pharmaceutical company.
IRB	Institutional Review Board, the US equivalent to an ethics committee.
MCT	multi-center trial, a trial that is carried out simultaneously following the same protocol at a number of different sites.
MIT	multiple independent trials, a series of trials conducted a number of sites following slightly varying methods, yet based on the same basic protocol which enables later inclusion in a meta analysis.

MPA — Medical Product Agency, the Swedish drug regulatory authority.

medical device — a medical technical device or aid.

meta analysis — literally an "after analysis," an analysis covering several differing studies that follow the same basic fundamentals and which are later combined and analyzed together.

monitor — person employed by the pharmaceutical company to be responsible that the study is conducted correctly.

NCE — New Chemical Entity, a drug with a new chemical structure.

NDA — New Drug Application, an application for registration of a drug in the USA.

PMS-study — Post-Marketing Surveillance study, a formalized follow up of a drug following registration in order to detect rare adverse reactions. Sometimes called a Phase V study.

per protocol analysis — an analysis using only those patients who completed the study according to the protocol.

pivotal study — a study with decisive impact on drug registration.

placebo — Latin: "I please"; an inactive substance or treatment.

principal investigator — the investigator bearing formal responsibility for an entire study, or at a clinic in a multi-center study.

protocol — a detailed description of a study's background, purpose, methodology, execution etc.

QA — Quality Assurance, an internal control undertaken by the pharmaceutical company.

randomization — random delegation to different treatment alternatives.

raw data — original data.

RDE — remote data entry, the direct entering of data from a study into a database, e.g., directly into a program in the investigator's computer, or similar.

run-in — period before beginning the treatment in which an effort is made to stabilize the patients' basic condition, such as when establishing a diagnosis.

SDV — source data verification, a control of the information in the CRF comparing directly to original data.

single blind — the patient is not aware of which treatment is being used.

SmPC — Summary of Product Characteristics, product information text approved by the authorities about a drug and continuing all information that a prescriber normally requires.

SOP — Standard Operating Procedures, written instructions about how certain tasks are to be conducted.

stratification — an assignment of patients into various [treatment] groups during randomization (in order to obtain an even distribution of a key characteristic among groups) or analysis (in order to study the effects in different groups).

source data — original data – notations in patient charts, EKG strips, X-rays etc. – sometimes called "raw data".

sponsor — an individual, company or institution taking responsibility for initiating, conducting and/or financing the study (according to the ICH GCP guidelines).

sub-investigator — investigator, a physician or dentist who participates in a clinical trial and bears the responsibility that the trial is conducted correctly, but lacks the formal head responsibility at the clinic in question. (cf. "co-investigator").

surrogate marker — Something measured instead of the actual phenomenon desired, is assumed to be an indicator for the same, and is usually easier or faster to measure. For example: arteriosclerosis in the carotid vessels as a surrogate marker for arteriosclerosis in the coronary vessel with subsequent myocardial infarction.

trial site — the site where the trial is conducted.

triple blind — neither the patient, investigator[s] nor person performing the analysis knows which treatment the patient received until after the final analysis has been performed.

wash-out — a period over which the previous treatment is discontinued, generally before start of the study treatment, or between different treatments in a study.

withdrawals — Patients who terminate a study on the advice of the investigator.

Appendix III – Declaration of Helsinki

Recommendations guiding medical physicians in biomedical research involving human subjects

Adopted by the 18th World Medical Assembly, Helsinki, Finland, June 1964, amended by the 29th World Medical Assembly, Tokyo, Japan, October1975, the 35th World Medical Assembly, Venice, Italy, October 1983 and the 41st World Medical Assembly, Hong Kong, September 1989 and the 48th General Assembly, Somerset West, Republic of South Africa, October 1996.

Introduction

It is the mission of the medical physician to safeguard the health of the people. His or her knowledge and consciense are dedicated to the fullfillment of this mission.

The declaration of Geneva of The World Medical Association binds the physician with the words, "The health of my patient will be my first consideration", and the International Code of Medical Ethics declares that, "A physician shall act only in the patient's interest when providing medical care which might have the effect of weakening the physical and mental condition of the patient".

The purpose of biomedical research involving human subjects must be to improve diagnostic, therapeutic and prophylactic procedures and the understanding of the aetiology and pathogenesis of disease.

In current medical practice most diagnostic, therapeutic and prophylactic procedures involve hazards. This applies especially to biomedical research.

Medical progress is based on research which ultimately must rest in part on experimentation involving human subjects.

In the field of biomedical research a fundamental distinction must be recognized between medical research in which the aim is essentially diagnostic or threrapeutic for a patient, and medical research, the essential object of of which is purely scientific and without direct diagnostic or therapeutic value to the person subjected to the research.

Special caution must be exercised in the conduct of research which may affect the environment, and the welfare of animals used for research must be respected.

Because it is essential that the results of laboratory experiments be applied to human beings to further scientific knowledge and to help suffering humanity the World Medical Association has prepared the following recommendations as a guide to every physician in biomedical research involving human subjects. They should be kept under review in the future. It must be stressed that the standards as drafted are only a guide to physicians all over the world. Physicians are not relieved from criminal, civil and ethical responsibilities under the laws of their own countries.

I. Basic principles

1. Biomedical research involving human subjects must conform to generally accepted scientific principles and should be based on adequately performed laboratory and animal expererimentation and on thorough knowledge of the scientific litterature.

2. The design and performance of each experimental procedure involving human subjects should be clearly formulated in an experimental protocol which should be transmitted for consideration, comment and guidance to a specially appointed committee independentof the investigator and the sponsor provided that this independent committe is in conformity with the laws and regulations in the country in which the research experiment is performed.

3. Biomedical research involving human subjects should be conducted only by scientifically qualified persons and under the supervision of a clinically competent person. The responsibility for the human subject must always rest with a medically qualified person and never rest on the subject of research, even though the subject has given his or her consent.

4. Biomedical research involving human subjects cannot legitimately be carried out unless the importance of the objective is in proportion to the inherent risk to the subject.

5. Every biomedical research project involving human subjects should be preceeded by careful assessment of predictable risks in comparison with foreseeable benefits to the subject or to others. Concern for the interests of the subject must always prevail over the interests of science and society.

6. The right of the research subject to safeguard his or her integrity must always be respected. Every precaution should be taken to respect the privacy of the subject and to minimize the impact of the study on the subjects physical and mental integrity and on the personality of the subject.

7. Physicians should abstain from engaging in research projects involving human subjects unless they are satisfied that the hazards involved are believed to be predictable. Physicians should cease any investigation if the hazards are found to outweigh the potential benefits.

8. In publication of the results of his or her research, the physician is obliged to preserve the accuracy of the results. Reports of experimentation not in accordance with the principles laid down in this Declaration should not be accepted for publication.

9. In any research on human beings, each potential subject must be adequately informed of the aims, methods, anticipated benefits and potential hazards of the study and the discomfort it may entail. He or she should be informed that he or she is at liberty to abstain from participation in the study and that he or she is free to withdraw his or her consent to participation at any time. The physician should then obtain the subjects freely-given informed consent, preferably in writing.

10. When obtaining informed consent for the research project the physician should be particularly cautious if the subject is in a dependent relationship to him or her or may consent under duress. In that case the informed consent should be obtained by a physician who is not engaged in the investigation and who is completely independent of this official relationship.

11. In the case of legal incompetence, informed consent should be obtained from the legal guardian in accordance with national legislation. Where physical or mental incapacity makes it impossible to obtain informed consent, or when the subject is a minor, permission from the responsible relative replaces that of the subject in accordance with national legislation.

10. Whenever the minor child is in fact able to give a consent, the minor's consent must be obtained in addition to the consent of the minor's legal guardian.

12. The research protocol should always contain a statement of the ethical considerations involved and should indicate that the principles enunciated in the present Declaration are complied with.

II. Medical research combined with profesional care (clinical research)

1. In the treatment of the sick person, the physician must be free to use a new diagnostic and therapeutic measure, if in his or her judgment it offers hope of saving life, reestablishing health or alleviating suffering.

2. The potential benefits, hazards and discomfort of a new method should be weighed against the advantages of the best current diagnostic and therapeutic methods.

3. In any medical study, every patient – including those of a control group – should be assured of the best proven diagnostic and therapeutic method. This does not exclude the use of inert placebo in studies where no proven diagnostic or therapeutic method exists.

4. The refusal of the patient to participate in a study must never interfere with the physician-patient relationship.

5. If the physician considers it essential not to obtain informed consent, the specific reason for this proposal should be stated in the experimental protocol for transmission to the independent committee (1,2).

6. The physician can combine medical research with professional care, the objective being the acquisition of new medical knowledge, only to the extent that medical research is justified by its potential diagnostic or therapeutic value for the patient.

III. Non-therapeutic biomedical research involving human subjects (Non-clinical biomedical research)

1. In the purely scientific application of medical research carried out on a human being, it is the duty of the physician to remain the protector of the life and health of that person on whom biomedical research is being carried out.

2. The subjects should be volunteers – either healthy persons or patients for whom the experimental design is not related to the patient's illness.

3. The investigator or the investigating team should discontinue the research if in his/her or their judgment it may, if continued, be harmful to the individual.

4. In research on man, the interest of science and society should never take precedence over considerations related to the well-being of the subject.

Index